Atlas of Male Genital Disorders

Giuseppe Micali • Marco Cusini •
Pompeo Donofrio • Franco Dinotta

Atlas of Male Genital Disorders

A Useful Aid for Clinical Diagnosis

Springer

Giuseppe Micali Dermatology Unit, Dipartimento di Specialità Medico-Chirurgiche, AOU "Policlinico-Vittorio Emanuele", Presidio "G. Rodolico", Catania, Italy

Marco Cusini Center for Sexually Transmitted Diseases, Dermatology Unit, Dipartimento di Anestesiologia, Terapia Intensiva e Scienze Dermatologiche, Fondazione IRCCS Ca' Granda, Ospedale Maggiore Policlinico, Milan, Italy

Pompeo Donofrio School of Dermatology and Venereology, "Federico II" University of Naples, Naples, Italy

Franco Dinotta Center for Sexually Transmitted Diseases, Dermatology Unit, Dipartimento di Specialità Medico-Chirurgiche, AOU "Policlinico-Vittorio Emanuele", Presidio "G. Rodolico", Catania, Italy

ISBN 978-88-470-2786-2 ISBN 978-88-470-2787-9 (eBook)

DOI 10.1007/978-88-470-2787-9

Springer Milan Dordrecht Heidelberg London New York
Library of Congress Control Number: 2012951967

9 8 7 6 5 4 3 2 1 2012 2013 2014 2015

Cover design: Ikona S.r.l., Milan, Italy
Typesetting: Ikona S.r.l., Milan, Italy

Springer-Verlag Italia S.r.l., Via Decembrio 28, I-20137 Milan
Springer is a part of Springer Science+Business Media (www.springer.com)

Preface

Male genital disorders encompass many aspects of gender medicine, including sexually transmitted infections and penile cancer. Since its inception as a specialty, dermatology has focused so prominently on genital disorders that many dermatology societies and units bear the names "dermatovenereology" or "dermatology and venereology". Professors Giuseppe Micali (Catania), Marco Cusini (Milan), Pompeo Donofrio (Naples), and Franco Dinotta (Catania) are well suited to act as learned authorities on genital disorders, as is clear from this skillfully crafted and extraordinarily useful compendium, the Atlas of Male Genital Disorders. All four of these distinguished physician-scientists have worked on genital disorders for many years. Each has actively participated in many scientific meetings on the subject and published papers in national and international journals. They run dedicated clinics on genital disorders at the Departments of Dermatology of the Universities of Milan, Naples, and Catania. The clinic in Catania is headed by the esteemed Professor Giuseppe Micali, an internationally acclaimed authority on penile lichen planus, penile cancer, and much more.

The editors and authors of this stellar work well deserve accolades as they have advanced and disseminated knowledge in this vital area of gender medicine. This erudite book merits the attention of practicing physicians worldwide, who will without doubt benefit from reading it.

October 2012 Robert A. Schwartz

Contents

Contributors

Piera Catalfo Dermatology Unit, AOU "Policlinico-Vittorio Emanuele", Presidio "G. Rodolico", Catania, Italy

Philip J. Cohen Department of Dermatology, UMDNJ - New Jersey Medical School, Newark, NJ, USA

Marco Cusini Center for Sexually Transmitted Diseases, Dermatology Unit, Dipartimento di Anestesiologia, Terapia Intensiva e Scienze Dermatologiche, Fondazione IRCCS Ca' Granda, Ospedale Maggiore Policlinico, Milan, Italy

Franco Dinotta Center for Sexually Transmitted Diseases, Dermatology Unit, Dipartimento di Specialità Medico-Chirurgiche, AOU "Policlinico-Vittorio Emanuele", Presidio "G. Rodolico", Catania, Italy

Paola Donofrio Dermatology and Venereology, "Federico II" University of Naples, Naples, Italy

Pompeo Donofrio School of Dermatology and Venereology, "Federico II" University of Naples, Naples, Italy

Salvatore Ferraro Dermatology Unit, AOU "Policlinico-Vittorio Emanuele", Presidio "G. Rodolico", Catania, Italy

Maria Grazia Francia Dermatology and Venereology, "Federico II" University of Naples, Naples, Italy

Francesco Lacarrubba Dermatology Unit, AOU "Policlinico-Vittorio Emanuele", Presidio "G. Rodolico", Catania, Italy

Giuseppe Micali Dermatology Unit, Dipartimento di Specialità Medico-Chirurgiche, AOU "Policlinico-Vittorio Emanuele", Presidio "G. Rodolico", Catania, Italy

Maria Letizia Musumeci Dermatology Unit, AOU "Policlinico-Vittorio Emanuele", Presidio "G. Rodolico", Catania, Italy

Maria Rita Nasca Dermatology Unit, AOU "Policlinico-Vittorio Emanuele", Presidio "G. Rodolico", Catania, Italy

Stefano Ramoni Center for Sexually Transmitted Diseases, Dermatology Unit, Dipartimento di Anestesiologia, Terapia Intensiva e Scienze Dermatologiche, Fondazione IRCCS Ca' Granda, Ospedale Maggiore Policlinico, Milan, Italy

Robert A. Schwartz Department of Dermatology, UMDNJ - New Jersey Medical School, Newark, NJ, USA

Anna Elisa Verzì Dermatology Unit, AOU "Policlinico-Vittorio Emanuele", Presidio "G. Rodolico", Catania, Italy

1 Anatomy of Male Genitalia

Franco Dinotta, Maria Rita Nasca, and Giuseppe Micali

F. Dinotta (✉)
Center for Sexually Transmitted Diseases
Dermatology Unit
Dipartimento di Specialità Medico-Chirurgiche
AOU "Policlinico – Vittorio Emanuele"
Presidio "G. Rodolico", Catania, Italy
e-mail: f.dinotta@unict.it

G. Micali et al., *Atlas of Male Genital Disorders*,
DOI: 10.1007/978-88-470-2787-9_1, © Springer-Verlag Italia 2013

Anatomy

Male genitalia include the penis and scrotum.

The penis is formed by two dorsal erectile structures (*corpora cavernosa*) and one ventral midline body (*corpus spongiosum*) which contains the urethra. These structures, covered by a thin and glabrous skin containing both apocrine and eccrine sweat glands, form the *shaft* of the penis. The corpus spongiosum is distally enlarged and rounded to form the *glans*, covered by semimucosa and topped by a vertical slit corresponding to the external *urethral meatus*. The base of the glans is called *corona* and it is proximally delimited by the *coronal sulcus* in which the secretion of freestanding balanopreputial sebaceous glands (*Tyson glands*) and epithelial debris, called *smegma*, may collect. The glans shows ventrally a linear cord, called *frenulum*, which extends from the urethral meatus to the coronal sulcus. When the frenulum is too short, erection may be painful and frenulotomy may be required. In uncircumcised men the glans is covered by a skin fold, called *prepuce* or *foreskin*. The foreskin is separated from the glans by a fold called *preputial sac*. The inner foreskin (semimucosa) is separated from the outer foreskin (skin) by a virtual boundary, the *preputial ring*, which may be narrowed as a result of inflammatory genital disorders, causing phimosis. A longitudinal line, corresponding to the area of conjunction during embryonal development (*median raphe*), is evident on the skin of the midventral shaft. The median raphe may be clearly raised or hyperpigmented in some subjects.

The scrotum is a sac, located below the shaft and between the inguinal folds, that contains the testicles that are attached to the deferent ducts. It is medially divided into two virtual cavities separated by an internal septum that corresponds, on the scrotal surface, to a skin groove called the *scrotal raphe*. The skin of the scrotum is usually thin and elastic and, in adults, it is pigmented and covered by hairs. It also contains both sweat (eccrine and apocrine) and sebaceous glands.

Male genitalia, especially the penis, have a rich vascularization and innervation.

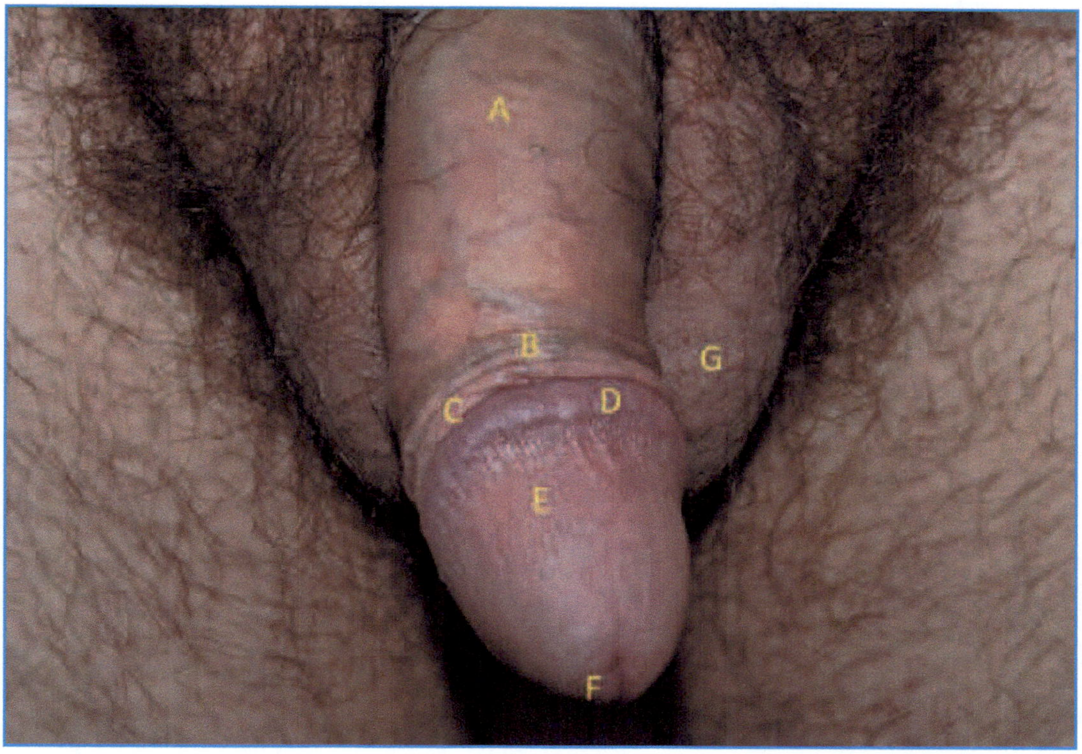

Fig. 1.1 Dorsal appearance of male genitalia. *A* Penile shaft. *B* Foreskin. *C* Coronal sulcus. *D* Corona. *E* Glans. *F* Urethral meatus. *G* Scrotum

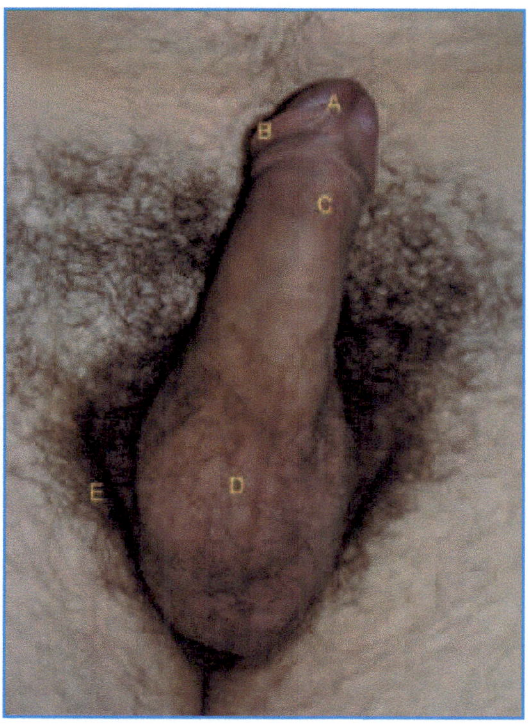

Fig. 1.2 Ventral appearance of male genitalia. *A* Frenulum. *B* Foreskin. *C* Penile median raphe. *D* Scrotal median raphe. *E* Inguinal fold

2 Infections

Marco Cusini, Stefano Ramoni, Salvatore Ferraro,
and Franco Dinotta

M. Cusini (✉)
Center for Sexually Transmitted Diseases
Dermatology Unit
Dipartimento di Anestesiologia, Terapia Intensiva e Scienze Dermatologiche
Fondazione IRCCS Ca' Granda
Ospedale Maggiore Policlinico, Milan, Italy
e-mail: m.cusini@policlinico.mi.it

G. Micali et al., *Atlas of Male Genital Disorders*,
DOI: 10.1007/978-88-470-2787-9_2, © Springer-Verlag Italia 2013

Genital Warts

Definition: Genital Warts (GW) are viral infections that affect the genital and perigenital area and seldom if ever evolve into cancer.

Etiology: GW are caused by some genotypes of Human Papilloma Virus (HPV), a DNA virus. In most cases infection follows sexual contact and it is a sexually transmitted disease. Low-risk HPV 6 and 11 are common causative agents, with a high efficacy of transmission (about 80%) and, fortunately, poor or no oncogenic potential. High-risk HPV 16 and 18 account for a low transmission percentage.

Epidemiology: genital HPV infection is very common; GW are the most frequent sexually transmitted infection in the Western world. Men and women are equally affected. GW are frequently encountered from age 20 to 45.

Clinical appearance: GW are clinically characterized by raised papular lesions that may become confluent (condyloma acuminatum). GW may be skin-coloured, pink, or brown, and may occur as verrucous lesions with a typical cauliflower appearance, or as papillomatous lesions (plaque or pedunculated lesions). Giant GW, also called Buschke-Löwenstein tumors, are uncommon. GW frequently develop on the foreskin and at the coronal sulcus and on the shaft and glans, but they may also extend to the urethral meatus and urethra.

Clinical course: after infection, HPV can remain clinically silent or induce the onset of visible lesions that can progress in number and size, remain stable or spontaneously disappear. HPV infection by high risk oncogenic HPVs may cause the development of genital malignancy.

Diagnosis: in the great majority of cases, diagnosis is based exclusively on clinical observation and past medical history. The use of acetic acid to enhance detection of subclinical infection is limited by its low specificity. Histology should be reserved to selected cases, such as immune-suppressed patients. Nuclear Antigen Amplification Technique (NAAT) is of no use in the routine clinical management of GW. Dermatoscopy may be helpful in the evaluation of initial or equivocal lesions; it shows, in papular lesions, a whitish network circumscribing areas centered by dilated glomerular vessels (*mosaic pattern*), and, in cauliflower-like lesions, irregular whitish projections arising from a common base and comprising elongated and dilated vessels (*finger-like pattern*).

Therapy: lesions may spontaneously regress in immunocompetent patients. The aim of therapy is to treat visible lesions and reduce the risk for sexual transmission. Therapeutic tools are usually divided into patient-applied (PA) and health care provider-applied (HCPA) methods. Of the former, imiquimod 5% cream and podophyllotoxin 0.15% cream are suggested in European and American guidelines. Of the HCPA methods, thermocautery, trichloroacetic acid, laser, and surgery are widely used.

Suggested Reading

Dall'Oglio F, D'Amico V, Nasca MR, Micali G (2012) Treatment of cutaneous warts: an evidence-based review. Am J Clin Dermatol 13:73-96

Dunne EF, Friedman A, Datta SD et al (2011) Updates on human papillomavirus and genital warts and counseling messages from the 2010 Sexually Transmitted Diseases Treatment Guidelines. Clin Infect Dis 53(Suppl 3):S143-52

Lacarrubba F, Dinotta F, Nasca MR, Micali G (2012) Enhanced diagnosis of genital warts with videodermatoscopy: histopatologic correlation. G Ital Dermatol Venereol 147:215-6

Lacey CJ, Woodhall SC, Wikstrom A, Ross J (2012) 2012 European guideline for the management of anogenital warts. J Eur Acad Dermatol Venereol [Epub ahead of print]

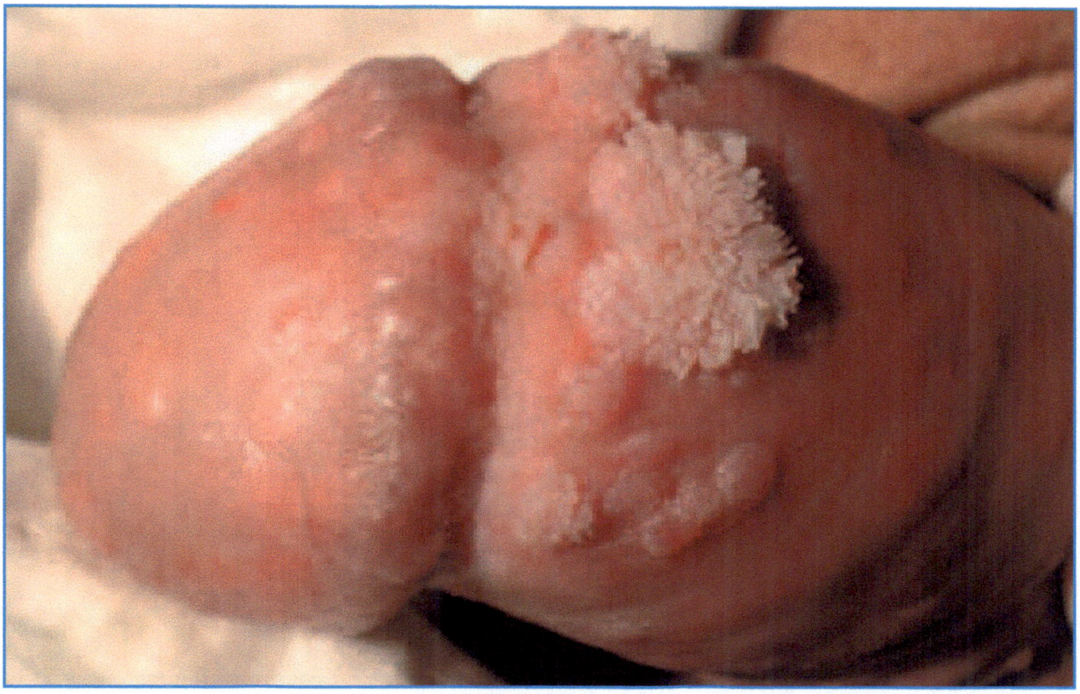

Fig. 2.1 Typical papular and papillomatous lesions on the foreskin

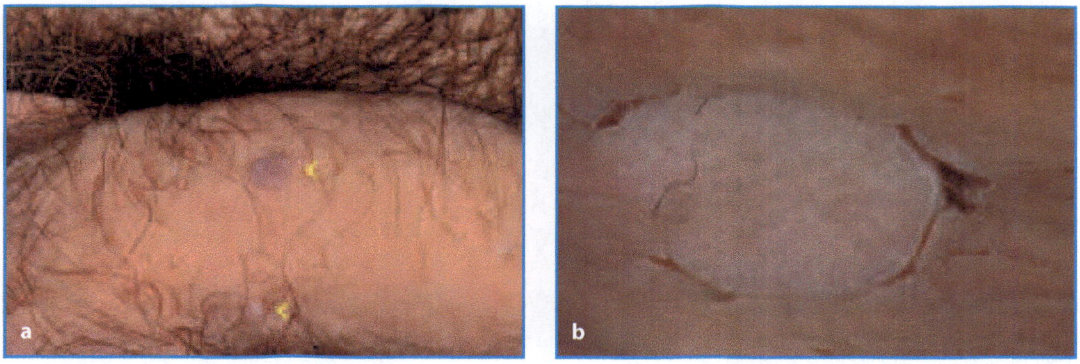

Fig. 2.2 Pinkish and flat papules on the shaft (**a**). **b** Videodermatoscopy (X10) of one lesion shows a whitish network circumscribing areas centered by dilated glomerular vessels (mosaic pattern)

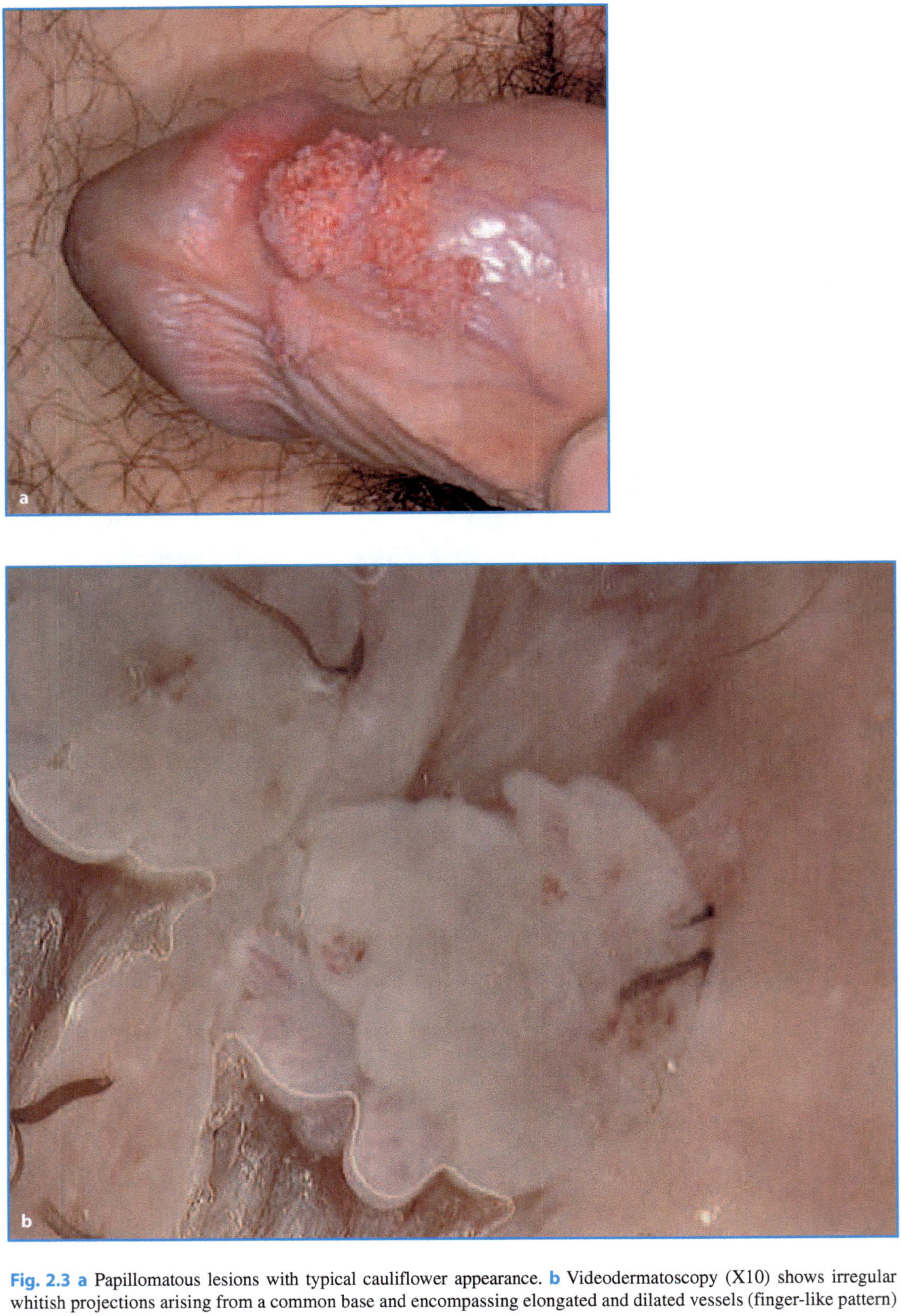

Fig. 2.3 **a** Papillomatous lesions with typical cauliflower appearance. **b** Videodermatoscopy (X10) shows irregular whitish projections arising from a common base and encompassing elongated and dilated vessels (finger-like pattern)

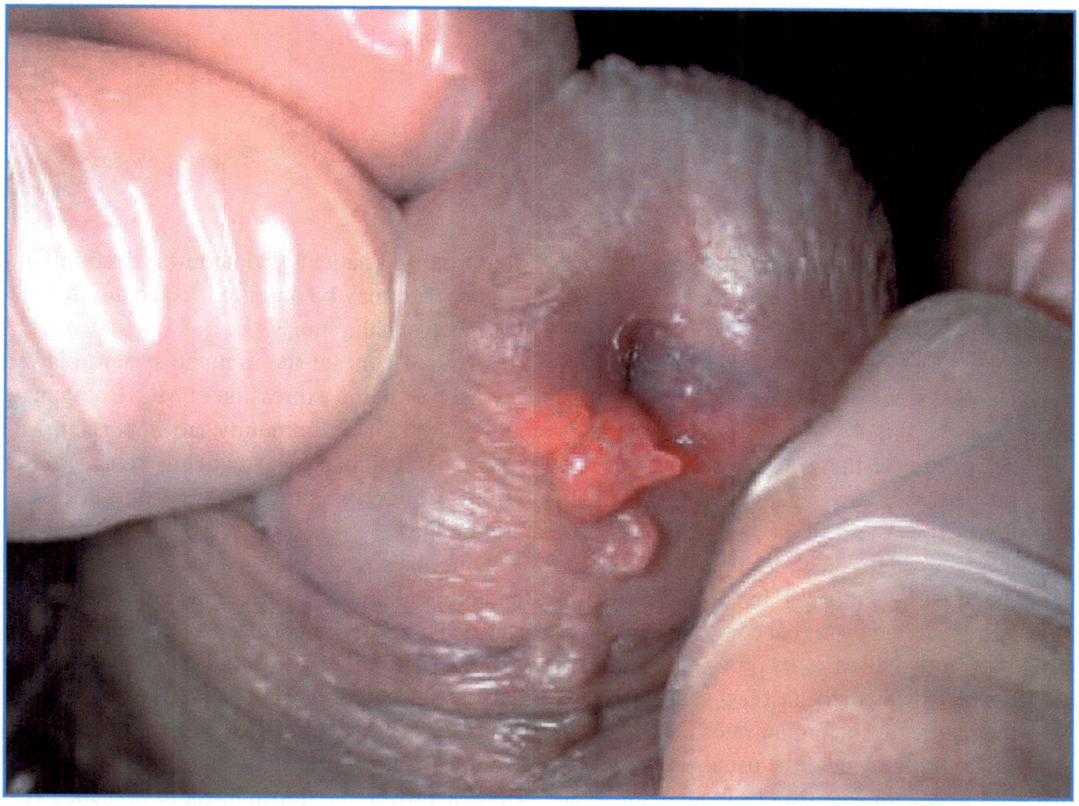

Fig. 2.4 Pedunculated lesion located in the urethra

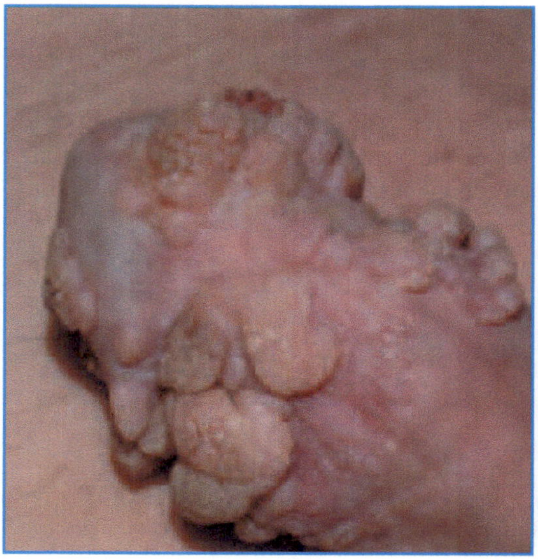

Fig. 2.5 Multiple lesions in an HIV+ patient

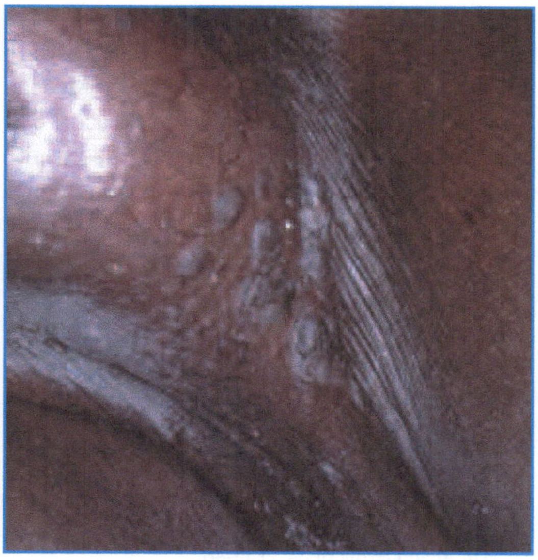

Fig. 2.6 Multiple and grayish papules on dark skin

Molluscum Contagiosum

Definition: Molluscum Contagiosum (MC) is a viral infection that may affect the genital and perigenital area.

Etiology: MC is caused by a poxvirus infection. The MC virus is a DNA virus able to persist latently on the skin.

Epidemiology: there are two peaks of frequency: the first in early age, with MC mostly located in the upper part of the body, and a second peak in young adults, with lesions located in the genital and perigenital area. In adults, MC is frequently transmitted by sexual contact and is a sexually transmitted disease. Its prevalence in adults has been increasing in the last few years. Men and women are affected at similar rates.

Clinical appearance: the usual appearance is that of an asymptomatic papule about 4 mm in diameter, white or skin-coloured, often showing a typical central umbilication. This depression, present in about one third of cases, is usually indicative of the disease. Genital lesions usually occur on the shaft and pubic area, although they may also be observed elsewhere. Usually, there are several lesions and in some cases as many as 50 MC can be observed. Lesions may sometimes reach 1 or 2 centimeters in diameter and may coalesce into large plaques. Giant MC are typical of immunocompromised patients. Sometimes, a red inflammatory halo may be observed, especially following mechanical traumas.

Clinical course: the immune system plays a pivotal role in the expression of MC. Both innate and cell-mediated immunity are important. MC runs a benign course. It frequently relapses after removal, but self-healing always occurs after several months.

Diagnosis: the clinical appearance is typical and other diagnostic procedures are seldom necessary. Histology can be used in atypical cases. In patients with AIDS, cryptococcosis may mimic MC lesions. Dermatoscopy shows a characteristic pattern consisting of a central polylobular white to yellow amorphous structure with a peripheral crown of reddish, linear or branched vessels, which do not usually cross the center of the lesion.

Therapy: the aim of therapy is to treat visible lesions and to reduce the risk of transmission through autoinoculation and sexual contact. Removal by curettage is a widely used and effective treatment. An anesthetic cream can be applied prior to removal. Self-healing is the rule in immunocompetent patients, but it may occur after several months.

Suggested Reading

Castronovo C, Lebas E, Nikkels-Tassoudji N, Nikkels AF (2012) Viral infections of the pubis. Int J STD AIDS 23:48-50

Micali G, Lacarrubba F, Massimino D, Schwartz RA (2011) Dermatoscopy: alternative uses in daily clinical practice. J Am Acad Dermatol 64:1135-46

Micali G, Lacarrubba F (2011) Augmented diagnostic capability using videodermatoscopy on selected infectious and non-infectious penile growths. Int J Dermatol 50:1501-5

Van Der Wouden JC, Van Der Sande R, Van Suijlekom-Smit LW et al (2009) Interventions for cutaneous molluscum contagiosum. Cochrane Database Syst Rev (4):CD004767

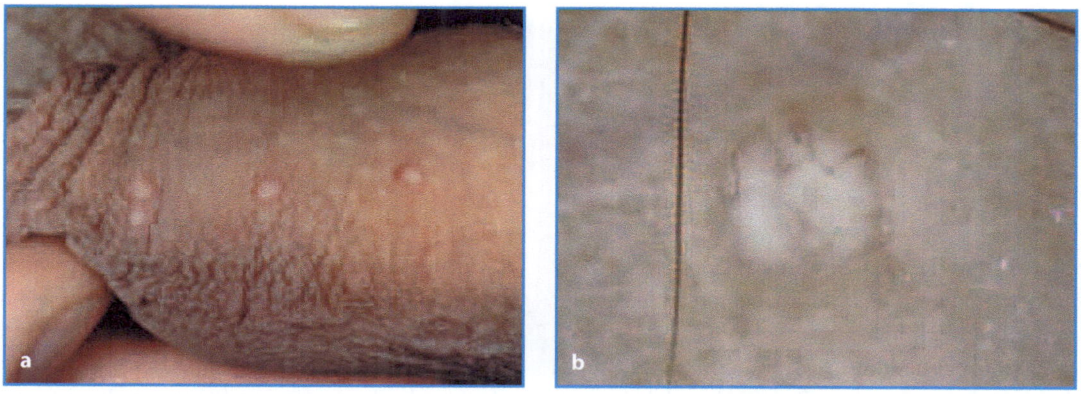

Fig. 2.7 a Skin-colored papules, with a characteristic central umbilication, located on the shaft. b Videodermatoscopy (X20) of a lesion shows a central yellow amorphous structure with a peripheral crown of reddish, linear vessels, which do not cross the center of the lesion

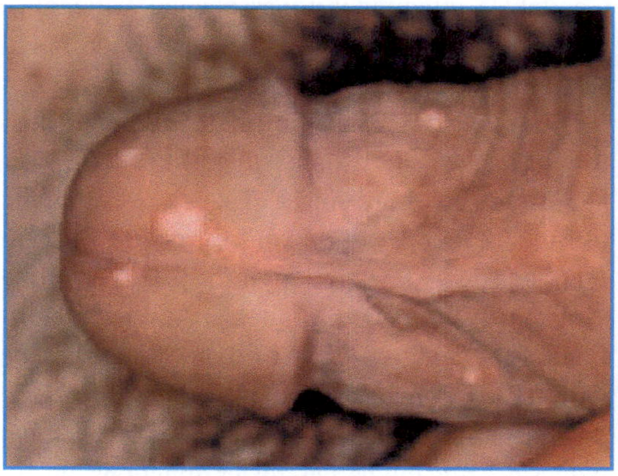

Fig. 2.8 Localization on the glans and shaft

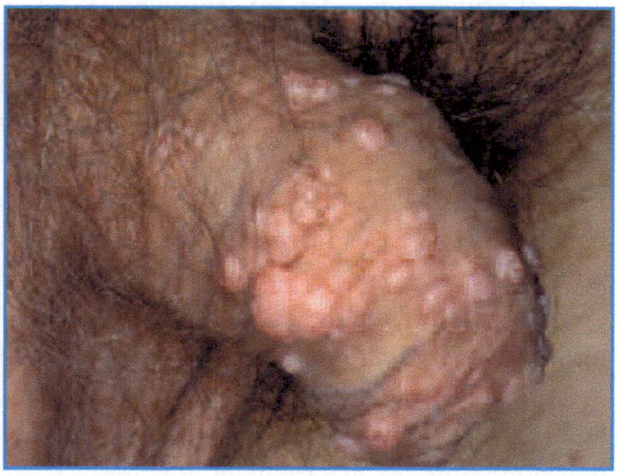

Fig. 2.9 Multiple papules and nodules, some of which of large diameter and confluent in plaques, in an HIV+ patient

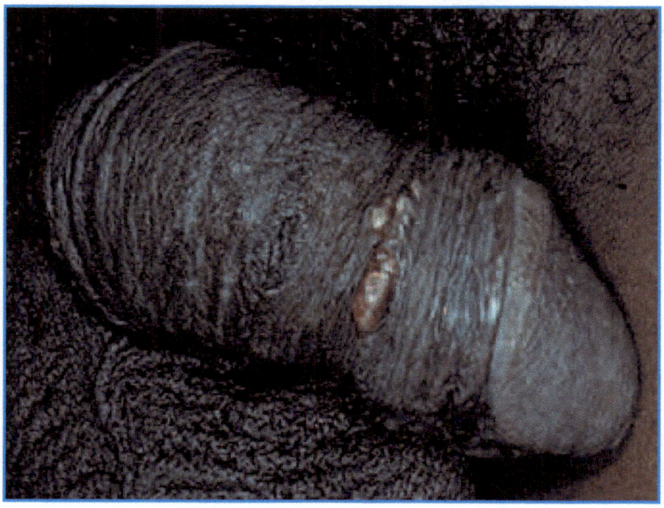

Fig. 2.10 Typical umbilicated papular lesions in an Afro-American patient

Herpes Simplex

Definition: Herpes Simplex (HS) is a sexually transmitted viral disorder that can reactivate after primary infection.

Etiology: genital HS is predominantly caused by the herpes virus type 2 (HSV2), a DNA virus. However, the frequency of herpes virus type 1 (HSV1) infection at genital sites has been progressively increasing in the last two decades, probably due to a change in sexual habits, and now almost 40% of primary episodes are caused by HSV1.

Epidemiology: sero-epidemiological studies show that HSV2 infection is widely spread, with a prevalence in the general population varying from 5% to 60%. Only about 25% of subjects infected with HSV2 develop recurrent disease. This percentage decreases in case of genital infection with HSV1.

Clinical appearance: primary HS is characterized by erythema with superimposed scattered and grouped vesicles, usually involving the glans and shaft. The lesions are often painful and general symptoms are also frequent. Recurrences are characterized by less severe lesions with involvement of smaller areas. The typical appearance of grouped vesicles is present in less than 50% of cases. Erosion of confluent blisters often results on policyclic shallow ulcerations. Atypical presentations include small crusted lesions or papules. Immunosuppressed patients exhibit atypical ulcers or hypertrophic lesions. HS may be associated with erythema multiforme, which recurs after each herpes outbreak.

Clinical course: after primary infection, which usually occurs through sexual contact, there is an incubation period of 7-10 days after which the clinical manifestations appear. After the primary infection heals, triggering factors such as fever, sun exposure, sexual intercourse, and hormonal fluctuations may promote recurrences of variable frequency and intensity. HSV1 produces milder genital lesions, with less common recurrences. Genital HS infection is not associated with malignancy, but it may increase the risk of additional sexually transmitted diseases.

Diagnosis: typical clinical features and history of recurrences usually suggest the correct diagnosis. A cytology smear (Tzanck test) may be useful, but it does not rule out varicella-zoster infection. The demonstration of the presence of the virus on swabs using the Nuclear Antigen Amplification Technique (NAAT) may sometimes be required in atypical presentations to confirm the diagnosis. Histology can be used in such cases, but it does not rule out herpes zoster infections, unless NAAT is performed on tissue samples.

Therapy: the aim of treatment is to induce lesion regression in the acute stage and to prevent frequent recurrences. Nucleoside analogues (oral acyclovir, valaciclovir, or famciclovir) are useful in reducing the severity and the duration of primary and recurrent outbreaks. Clinical resistance to these drugs is not an issue in immunocompetent patients, but it may sometimes be troublesome in immunocompromised subjects.

Suggested Reading

Dinotta F, De Pasquale R, Nasca MR et al (2009) Disseminated herpes simplex infection in a HIV+ patient. G Ital Dermatol Venereol 144:205-9

Gupta R, Warren T, Wald A (2007) Genital herpes. Lancet 370:2127-37

Martinez V, Caumes E, Chosidow O (2008) Treatment to prevent recurrent genital herpes. Curr Opin Infect Dis 21:42-8

Van Wagoner NJ, Hook EW 3rd (2012) Herpes diagnostic tests and their use. Curr Infect Dis Rep 14:175-84

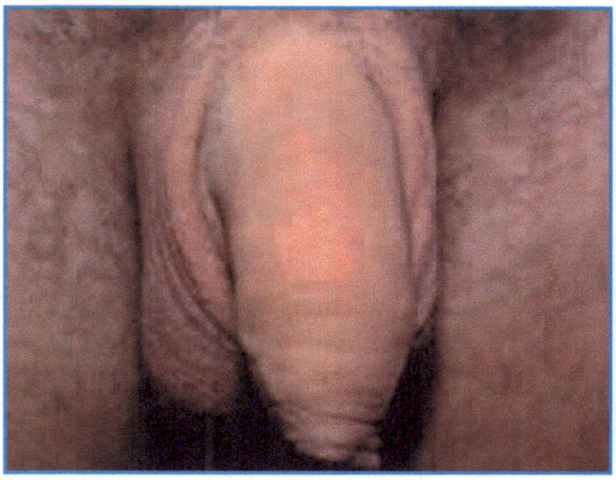

Fig. 2.11 Typical grouped vesicles on the shaft

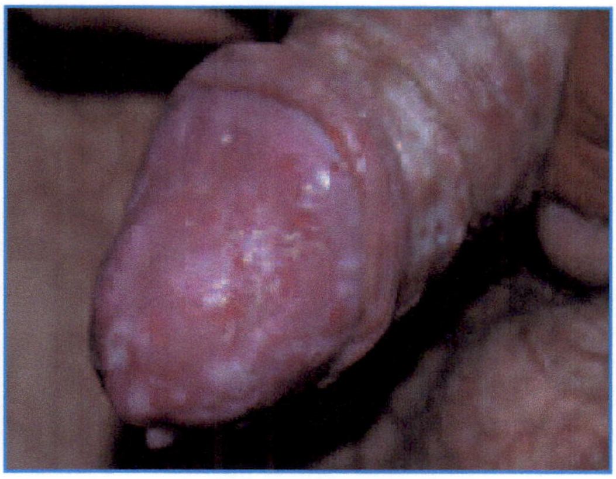

Fig. 2.12 Multiple vesicles on the glans

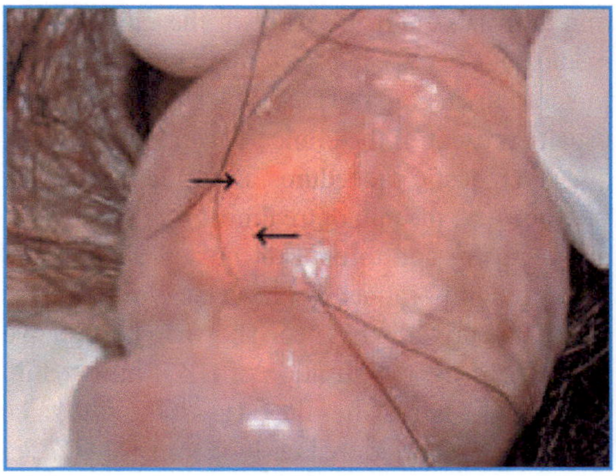

Fig. 2.13 Confluent and polycyclic (*arrows*) erosions on the inner foreskin

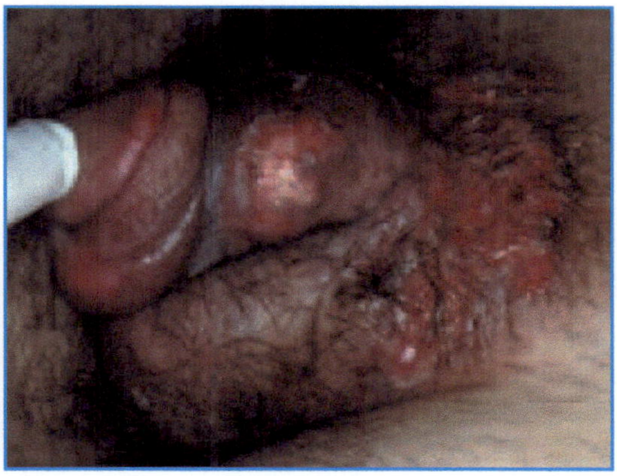

Fig. 2.14 Multiple erosions, ulcers, and edema in an HIV+ patient

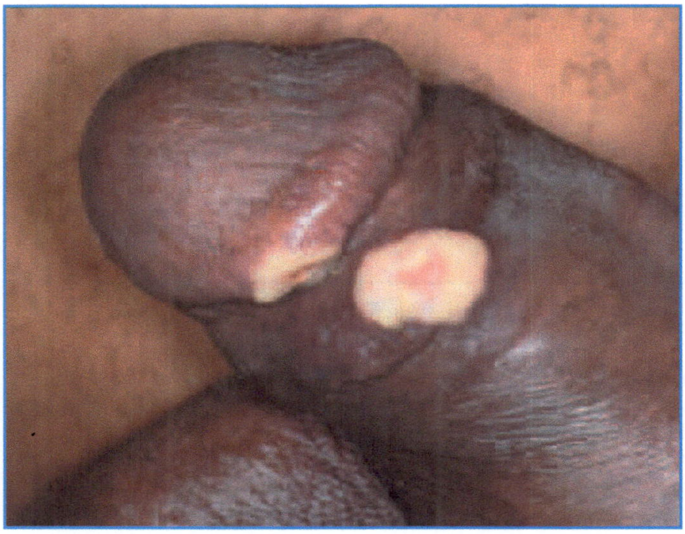

Fig. 2.15 Ulcerative lesions on the corona and foreskin in an HIV+ Afro-American patient

Herpes Zoster

Definition: Herpes Zoster (HZ) is due to a local recurrence of Varicella Zoster Virus (VZV) infection and it follows chickenpox after several years.

Etiology: after primary infection, the virus settles at the root of sensitive ganglia and from there spreads through the territory of innervation of a sensitive nerve whenever reactivation from a latent stage occurs.

Epidemiology: it has been reported that almost 30% of the general population develops HZ during their lifetime. Frequency increases with age, and incidence is much higher in immunosuppressed patients.

Clinical appearance: the usual appearance is that of vesicles exhibiting a typical unilateral localization, involving the area of distribution of a sensitive nerve ending (dermatome). Penile lesions may occur as the result of viral spread through the nervum pudendum. Immunosuppressed patients may develop distant lesions as the result of HZ dissemination.

Clinical course: HZ usually breaks out with local paresthesias or pain, followed after 24-48 hours by the onset of vesicles in the involved site. General symptoms are infrequent. Lesions progress for five-seven days and then start to heal, usually without scarring but with frequent residual hypo- or hyperpigmentation. Postherpetic neuralgia is a major complication, especially in the elderly. Unlike herpes simplex, HZ usually does not recur in immunocompetent patients.

Diagnosis: differential diagnosis of HZ involving the genital area includes herpes simplex infection. HZ occurs in a dermatomal unilateral distribution and it is more frequent in the elderly. Past medical history is negative for previous outbreaks. In addition, in case of HZ, extragenital lesions are usually present. If the clinical features are typical, other diagnostic procedures are seldom required.

Therapy: the aim of treatment is to speed clinical recovery and to control the associated pain. Therapy with oral acyclovir, valaciclovir, famciclovir, and brivudin has been shown to be effective on the severity and duration of HZ if initiated no later than 48 hours after the onset of the skin rash. It has been reported that early therapy of HZ can reduce the risk of postherpetic neuralgia. For this reason, prompt treatment is recommended in patients over the age of sixty. A vaccine has recently become available.

Suggested Reading

Dhiman N, Wright PA, Espy MJ et al (2011) Concurrent detection of herpes simplex and varicella-zoster viruses by polymerase chain reaction from the same anatomic location. Diagn Microbiol Infect Dis 70:538-40

Schmader KE, Dworkin RH (2008) Natural history and treatment of herpes zoster. J Pain 9(Suppl 1):S3-9

Urman CO, Gottlieb AB (2008) New viral vaccines for dermatologic disease. J Am Acad Dermatol 58:361-70

Weinberg JM (2007) Herpes zoster: epidemiology, natural history, and common complications. J Am Acad Dermatol 57(Suppl 6):S130-5

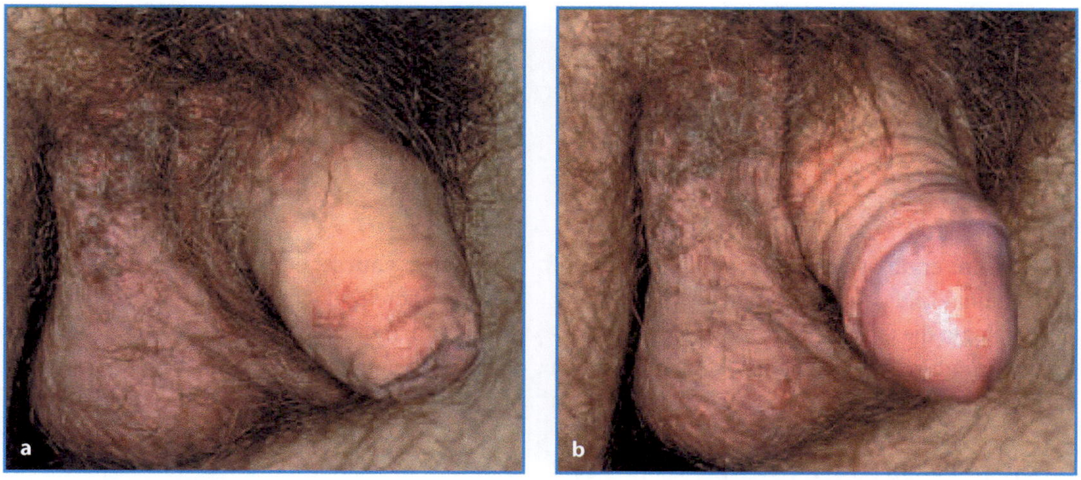

Fig. 2.16 Typical unilateral grouped vesicles involving the scrotum and the shaft (a), and the glans (b) in an HIV+ patient

Erythrasma

Definition: erythrasma is a bacterial infection of the inguinal folds.

Etiology: the infection is caused by *Corynebacterium minutissimum* (CM). Some conditions such as diabetes, obesity, and a moist environment can favor this disease.

Epidemiology: it has been reported that about 20% of the general population is colonized by CM. Erythrasma is more frequent in young males.

Clinical appearance: the usual appearance is that of small, well-demarcated, reddish or brownish maculae that increase in size and coalesce into larger patches. Lesions are smooth and may show a dusty scaling. The inguinal folds and proximal shaft of the penis are common locations, whereas the scrotum and penis are generally unaffected. Sometimes, small dotted lesions near the edges may suggest the diagnosis.

Clinical course: erythrasma is usually asymptomatic. Increased temperature, humidity, maceration, and friction can sometimes induce some itching. If untreated, the lesion tends to spread slowly involving large areas of the inner surface of the thighs. Recurrence after therapy is quite frequent.

Diagnosis: clinical diagnosis is usually straightforward. Wood's light examination is useful in making a differential diagnosis with tinea cruris, disclosing a characteristic coral-red fluorescence in erythrasma. CM may grow on special media but microbiology tests are seldom used. A biopsy is not generally performed.

Therapy: oral therapy with erythromycin, for 7 days, is effective, as is topical application of imidazole and of fusidic acid creams.

Suggested Reading

Avci O, Tanyildizi T, Kusku E (2011) A comparison between the effectiveness of erythromycin, single-dose clarithromycin and topical fusidic acid in the treatment of erythrasma. J Dermatolog Treat [Epub ahead of print]
Holdiness MR (2002) Management of cutaneous erythrasma. Drugs 62:1131-41
Holdiness MR (2003) Erythrasma and common bacterial skin infections. Am Fam Physician 67:254

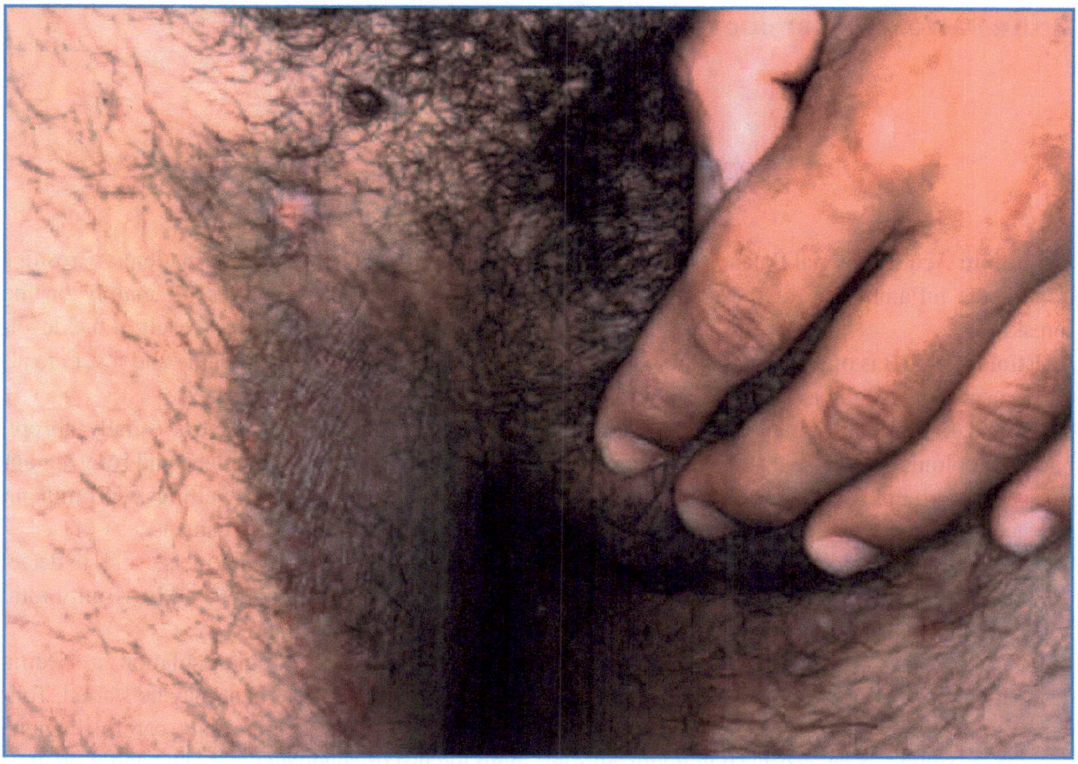

Fig. 2.17 Large, sharply demarcated, and brownish patch involving the inguinal folds

Acute Bacterial Balanoposthitis

Definition: Acute Bacterial Balanoposthitis (ABB) is an acute inflammation of the glans and inner foreskin.

Etiology: ABB is often secondary to other conditions, such as sexually transmitted urethritis, that cause maceration and irritation with subsequent bacterial colonization. Usually, a mixed infection is present, with both anaerobic and aerobic bacteria such as *Streptococcus* or *Staphylococcus*.

Epidemiology: epidemiological data are scant. ABB is more frequent in uncircumcised patients, although it may also occur in circumcised individuals.

Clinical appearance: several different features depicting specific clinical types of ABB have been described. Among these, *erosive balanoposthitis* is mainly due to anaerobia in association with non-treponematous spirochetes and it occurs almost exclusively in uncircumcised patients. Erosions and even ulceration are present, mainly on the glans. More severe cases may result in the development of gangrene. Adenopathy and fever are always present.

Clinical course: the onset is usually abrupt, with itching and pain. The glans and foreskin appear red and swollen. If swelling is prominent, phymosis or paraphymosis can ensue.

Diagnosis: a swab for culture is useful to detect the bacteria involved and to address antibiotic therapy.

Therapy: after microbial isolation, a specific systemic antibiotic treatment may be started. Topical treatment is also important: careful hygiene with the use of adequate detergents and mild antiseptics, and the application of creams or ointments, may lead to prompt improvement of the symptoms.

Suggested Reading

Cree GE, Willis AT, Phillips KD, Brazier JS (1982) Anaerobic balanoposthitis. Br Med J 284:859-60

Lincopan N, Neves P, Mamizuka EM, Levy CE (2010) Balanoposthitis caused by Pseudomonas aeruginosa co-producing metallo-beta-lactamase and 16S rRNA methylase in children with hematological malignancies. Int J Infect Dis 14:e344-7

Minami M, Wakimoto Y, Matsumoto M et al (2010) Characterization of Streptococcus pyogenes isolated from balanoposthitis patients presumably transmitted by penile-oral sexual intercourse. Curr Microbiol 61:101-5

Muratov ID (2004) Bacteriological pattern of acute purulent balanoposthitis in children. Zh Mikrobiol Epidemiol Immunobiol 2:83-5

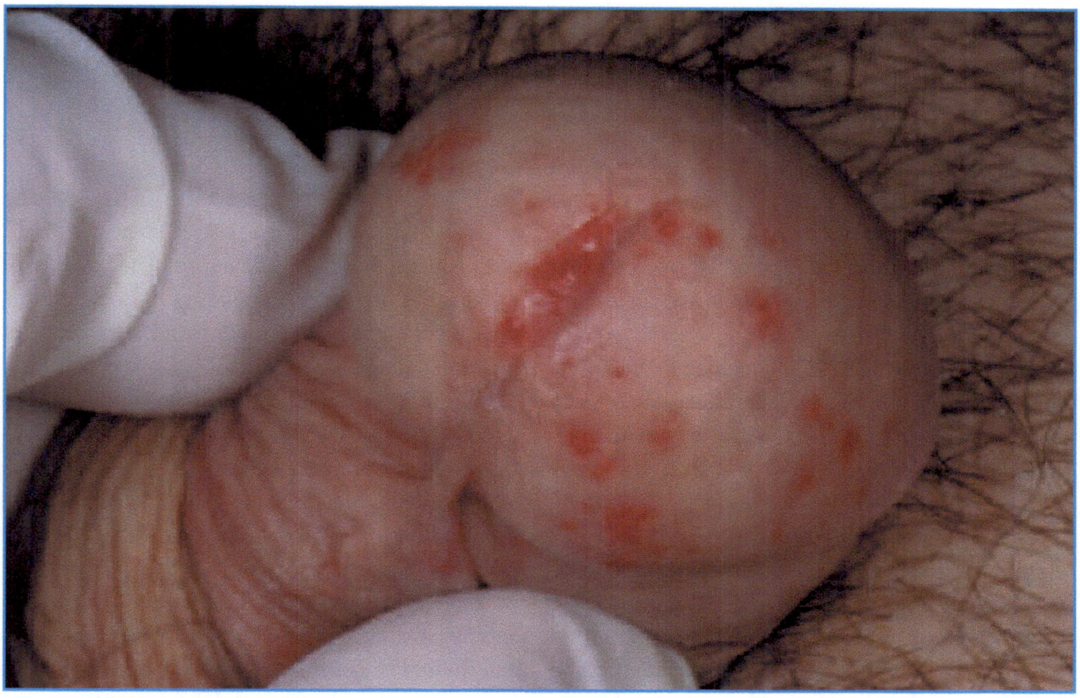

Fig. 2.18 Multiple and small erosions of the glans and the urethral meatus

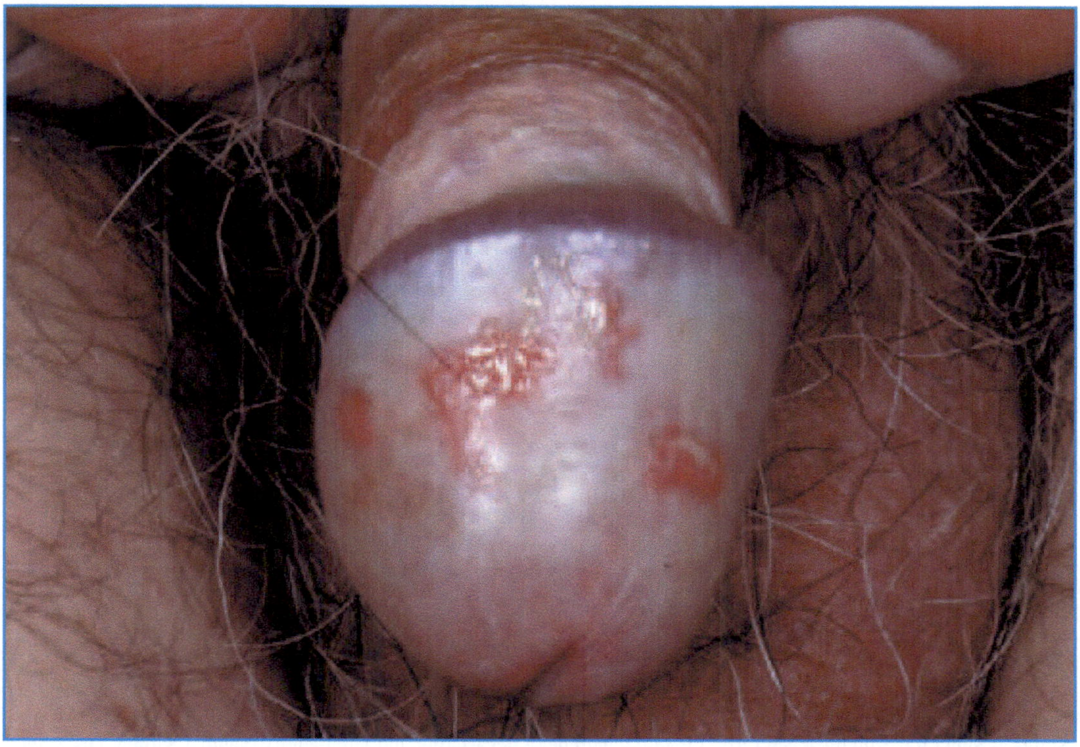

Fig. 2.19 Multiple erosions of the glans

Fournier's Gangrene

Definition: Fournier's gangrene is a necrotizing fasciitis developing on the genitalia and rapidly involving adjacent tissues.

Etiology: causative agents include many different microorganisms, either anaerobic, such as *Bacteroides fragilis*, or Gram +, such as beta-hemolytic *Streptococcus* group A, or Gram –, such as *Proteus* and *Enterococcus*. This condition is favored by local (urogenital surgery) and systemic (diabetes mellitus, hematological diseases) factors.

Epidemiology: it is rare.

Clinical appearance: Fournier's gangrene generally starts with a painful genital edema; the most frequent localization is the scrotum. The involved tissues rapidly become necrotic and fever with general symptoms develops. The severity of the disease may vary, depending on localization, rate of cutaneous involvement, and occurrence of generalized sepsis.

Clinical course: this is an acute condition with a mortality rate of 25%, due to sepsis and disseminated intravascular coagulation.

Diagnosis: final diagnosis should be confirmed by microbiological investigations identifying the causative agents.

Therapy: a broad-spectrum antibiotic therapy should be started as soon as possible and intensive care should be considered. Medical treatment must be associated with surgical debridement.

Suggested Reading

Fajdic J, Gotovac N, Hrgovic Z (2011) Fournier gangrene: our approach and patients. Urol Int 87:186-91

Jensen P, Zachariae C, Grønhøj Larsen F (2010) Necrotizing soft tissue infection of the glans penis due to atypical Candida species complicated with Fournier's gangrene. Acta Derm Venereol 90:431-2

Singh V, Sinha RJ, Sankhwar SN (2011) Penile gangrene: a devastating and lethal entity. Saudi J Kidney Dis Transpl 22:359-61

Talwar A, Puri N, Singh M (2010) Fournier's gangrene of the penis: a rare entity. J Cutan Aesthet Surg 3:41-4

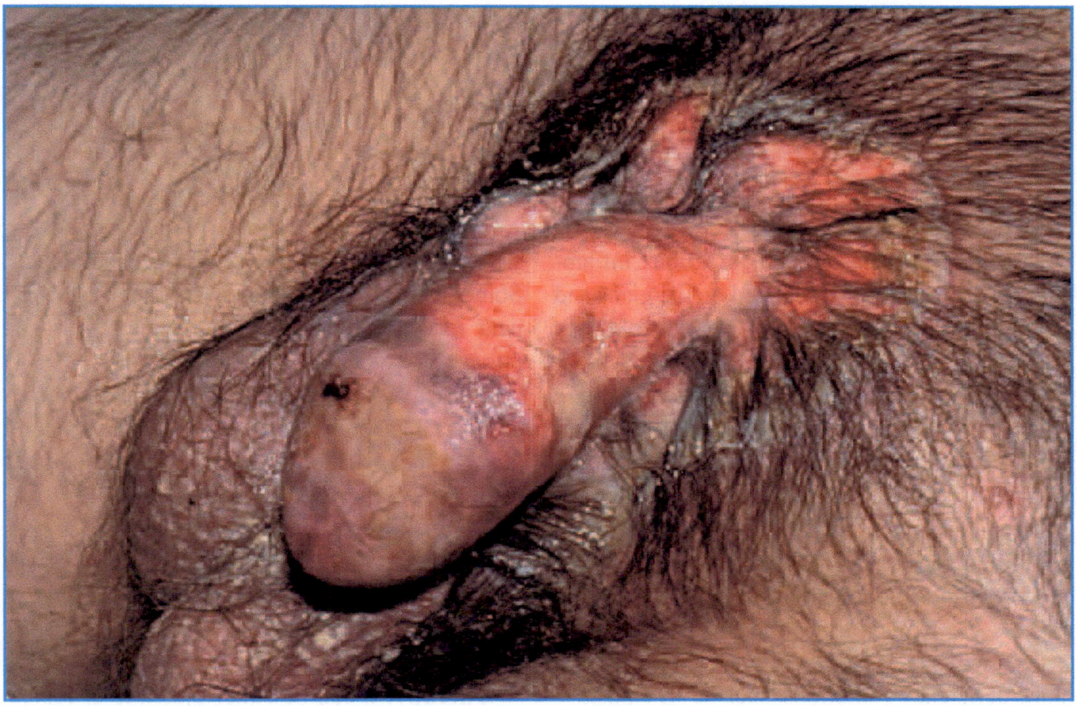

Fig. 2.20 Extensive ulcero-necrotic lesions in an HIV+ patient

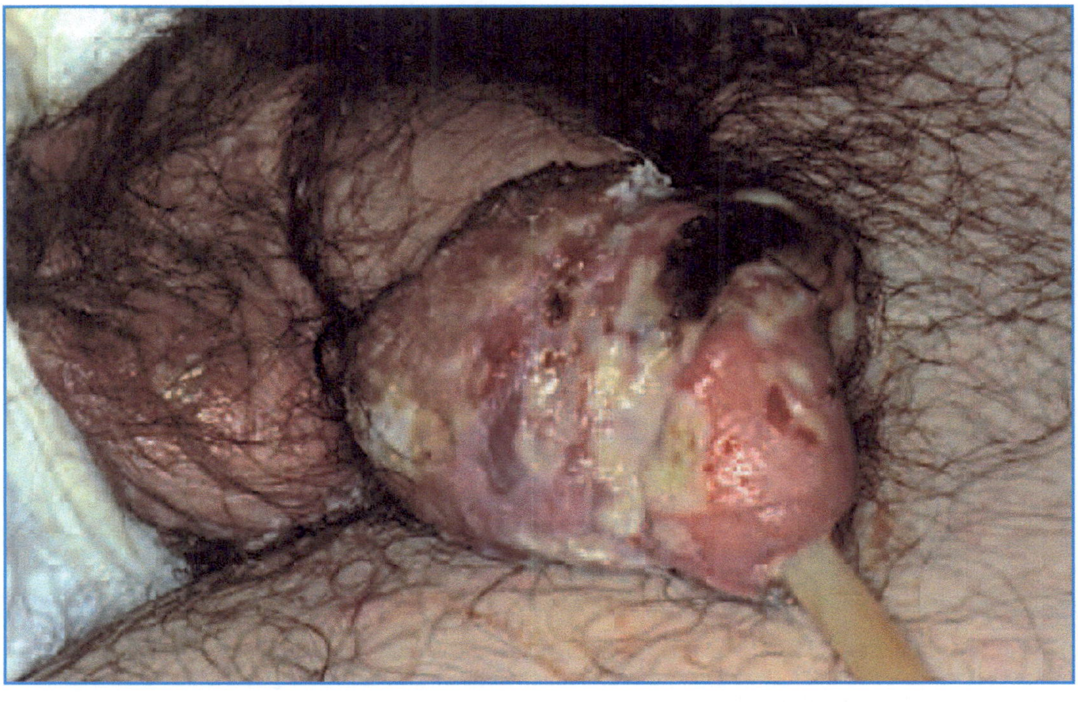

Fig. 2.21 Ulcero-necrotic lesions involving the penis and the scrotum in an HIV+ patient

Candidiasis

Definition: candidiasis is an infectious inflammatory disease usually localized on the glans and on the inner foreskin, but the inguinal fold may also be involved.

Etiology: candidiasis is caused by *Candida sp.*, which are almost always present in the vaginal flora but infrequent on male genitalia. Under some circumstances *Candida sp.* can colonize the glans and coronal sulcus and cause an inflammation. It may be sexually transmitted.

Epidemiology: it is more frequent in diabetic patients but it may also affect male partners of women with chronic or recurrent candidiasis. Immune deficiency conditions, such as HIV positivity, chronic topical steroid therapy, or systemic treatment with chemotherapeutic agents and other immune active drugs are often associated.

Clinical appearance: the first appearance is that of numerous white pustules or red macules with desquamative borders spotted on the glans. Sometimes the whole glans and coronal sulcus appear red and shiny with small yellow pustules (strawberry glans).

Clinical course: the onset of genital candidiasis is acute. It generally self-heals in 4-5 days, but relapses after sexual contacts with infected partners are the rule.

Diagnosis: the clinical appearance may suggest the correct diagnosis. KOH examination shows the presence of hyphae and sporae typical of *Candida sp.* Culture can be helpful to identify the species involved.

Therapy: it can be either systemic or topical with azole derivatives. In young adults, antiseptics are often enough to achieve healing. Whenever possible, the treatment should be prescribed to the patient and to his partners.

Suggested Reading

Aridogan IA, Izol V, Ilkit M (2011) Superficial fungal infections of the male genitalia: a review. Crit Rev Microbiol 37:237-44

Dockerty WG, Sonnex C (1995) Candidal balano-posthitis: a study of diagnostic methods. Genitourin Med 71:407-9

Lisboa C, Ferreira A, Resende C, Rodrigues AG (2009) Infectious balanoposthitis: management, clinical and laboratory features. Int J Dermatol 48:121-4

Mayser P (1999) Mycotic infections of the penis. Andrologia 31(Suppl 1):13-6

Waugh MA (1998) Balanitis. Dermatol Clin 16:757-62

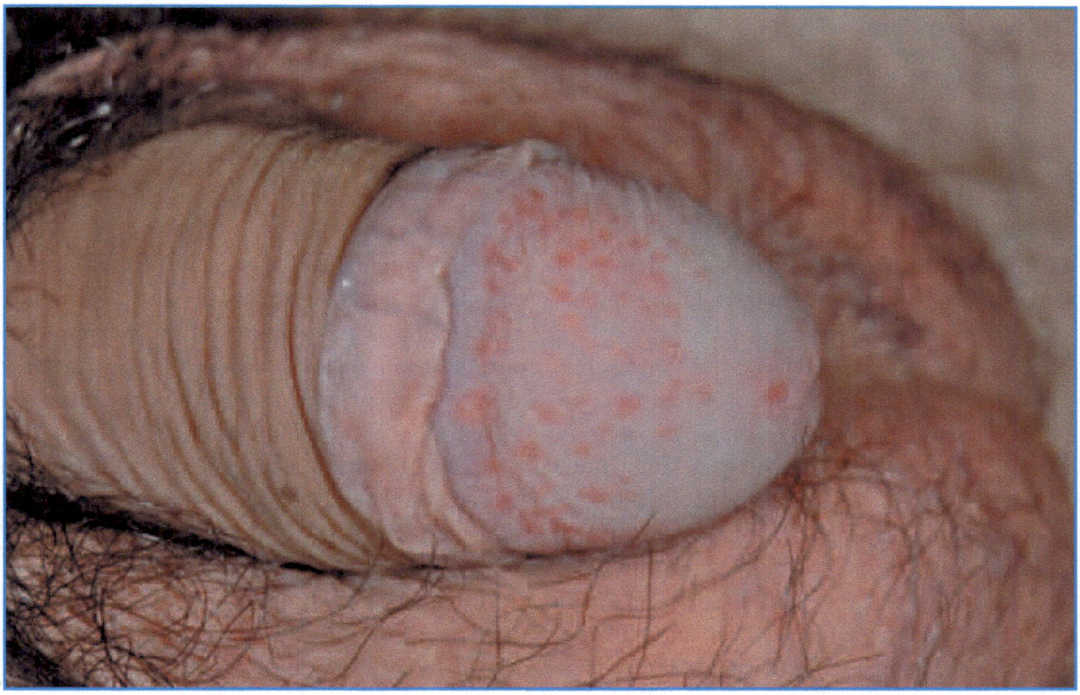

Fig. 2.22 Multiple small red macules on the glans

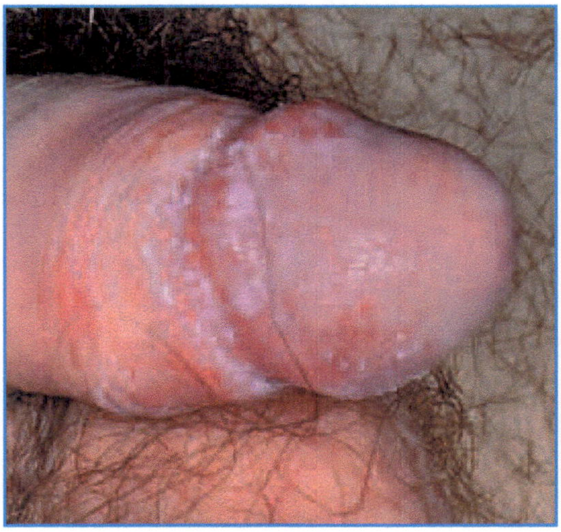

Fig. 2.23 Erythematous lesions and whitish discharge on the glans and foreskin

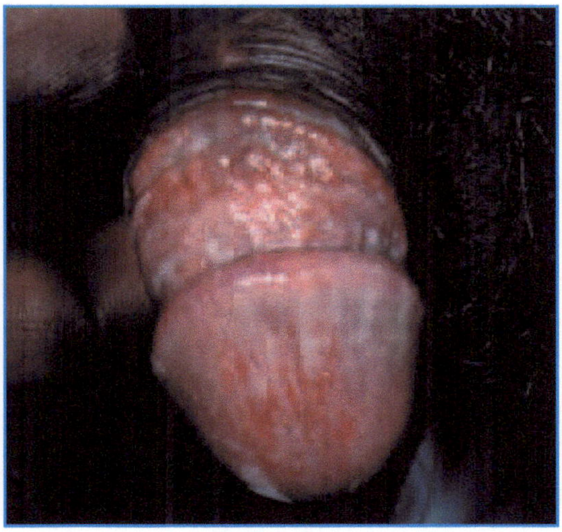

Fig. 2.24 Intense erythema and whitish discharge on the glans and foreskin in an Afro-American patient

Tinea Cruris

Definition: Tinea Cruris (TC) is a fungal infection that usually involves the inguinal fold and may extend to the genitalia.

Etiology: TC is caused by dermatophytes. *Epidermophyton floccosum* is the most frequent etiological agent, but others (*Trichophyton rubrum*, *Trichophyton mentagrophytes*) may be involved.

Epidemiology: the disease is mainly observed in postpubertal men, and men are in general more affected than women. It is rare in childhood.

Clinical appearance: TC starts from one inguinal fold with red circular or half-moon shaped lesions with desquamative borders that grow centrifugally and involve the contralateral fold. Erythematous papules and pustules may occur, especially within the leading edge. TC generally does not extend to the scrotum and/or penis unless the patient is immunosuppressed. When the disease affects the penis, it usually appears as a round, itchy lesion, with a scaling border. Inappropriate treatment with topical corticosteroid may cause the development of tinea incognita, e.g. a misdiagnosed atypical fungal infection.

Clinical course: usually, TC is eradicated with therapy. However, recurrences may occur, so that affected patients may require the ongoing use of topical antimycotic therapy to prevent relapses.

Diagnosis: a clinical diagnosis made on the peripheral scaling must be confirmed by microscopic diagnosis and/or culture.

Therapy: topical antifungal creams (azoles, allylamines) applied for two weeks are usually effective. Extensive forms may require oral antifungal therapy.

Suggested Reading

Pandey SS, Chandra S, Guha PK et al (1981) Dermatophyte infection of the penis. Association with a particular undergarment. Int J Dermatol 20:112-4
Pielop J, Rosen T (2001) Penile dermatophytosis. J Am Acad Dermatol 44:864-7
Romano C, Ghilardi A, Papini M (2005) Nine male cases of tinea genitalis. Mycoses 48:202-4

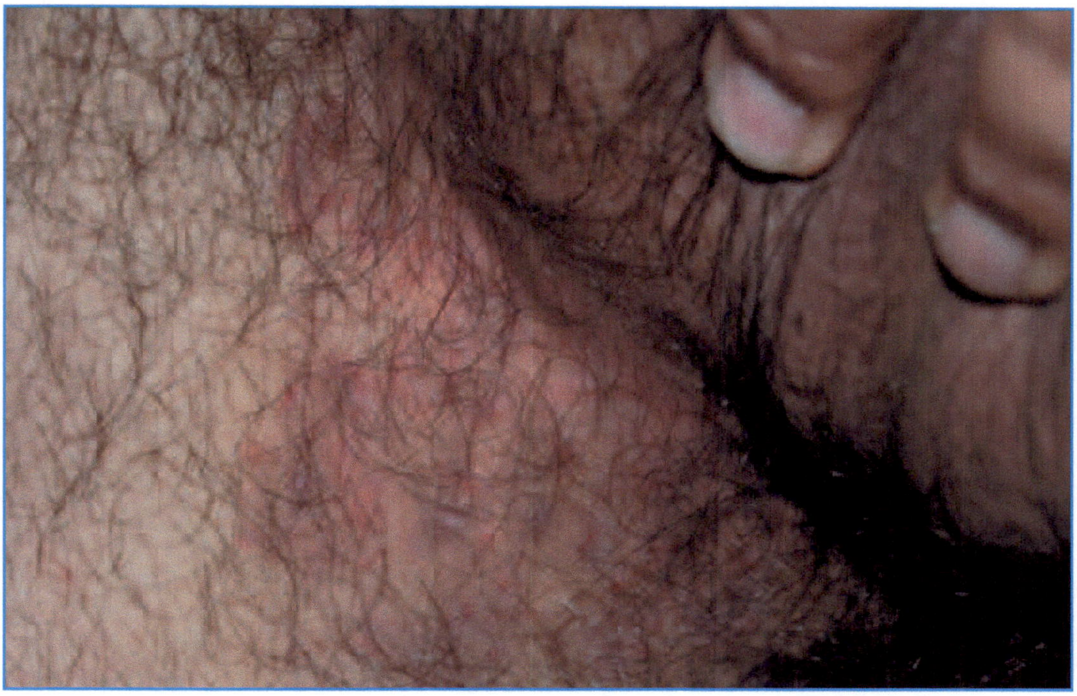

Fig. 2.25 Scaling, sharply-marginated, and reddish patch involving the groin

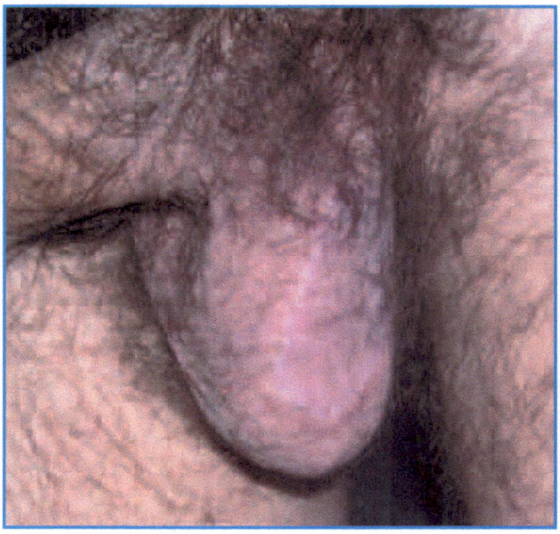

Fig. 2.26 Roundish patch, with typical scaling border, on the scrotum

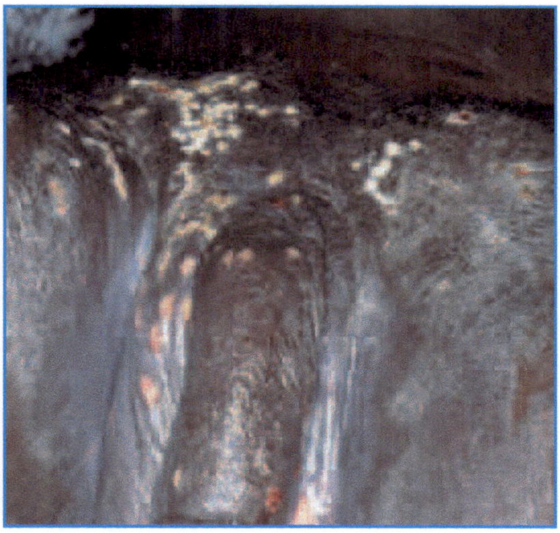

Fig. 2.27 Multiple, confluent, grayish, and scaling patches involving the penis, the scrotum and the groins in an Afro-American patient

3 Infestations

Marco Cusini, Francesco Lacarrubba, Stefano Ramoni, and Franco Dinotta

M. Cusini (✉)
Center for Sexually Transmitted Diseases
Dermatology Unit
Dipartimento di Anestesiologia, Terapia Intensiva e Scienze Dermatologiche
Fondazione IRCCS Ca' Granda
Ospedale Maggiore Policlinico, Milan, Italy
e-mail: m.cusini@policlinico.mi.it

G. Micali et al., *Atlas of Male Genital Disorders*,
DOI: 10.1007/978-88-470-2787-9_3, © Springer-Verlag Italia 2013

Pubic Lice

Definition: pubic lice represent a cutaneous parasitosis characterized by itching and by the presence of insects and/or their nits in the pubic hair.

Etiology: pubic lice are insects called *Phthirus pubis*. After parasitation, the female insects, firmly attached to pubic hairs, deliver their nits which unfold after 6-8 days. *Phthirus pubis* is an emathophagous insect, and itching is caused by its bites. The ectoparasitosis is usually spread by intimate or sexual contact with an infested person. Contamination may also occur indirectly (underwear, bedclothes). It is classified as a sexually transmitted disease.

Epidemiology: pubic lice are very common, and the disorder occurs worldwide. Accurate data are difficult to collect because pubic lice infestations are not considered a reportable condition by many governments.

Clinical appearance: the patient complains of itching in the pubic area. Physical examination reveals the presence of the insects and/or their nits attached to pubic hairs. Skin lesions resulting from scratching and *maculae caeruleae* from the insect bites may be found on the genital skin, and tiny blood spots may often be detected in the patient's underwear.

Clinical course: the disease starts in the pubic area but it can extend to other hair-rich sites such as trunk, axillae and lashes. In male patients it may also extend to the trunk.

Diagnosis: the clinical presentation is generally indicative of the diagnosis. Videodermatoscopy easily ensures a detailed identification of both mites and nits. Full, viable nits appear as opaque structures, with a rounded free ending, fixed to the hair shaft; empty nits appear as translucent structures with a flat and fissured free ending.

Therapy: effective treatment is based on the use of topical insecticides, such as permethrin 1% cream applied to the affected area and washed off after 10 minutes. Another application after 10 days is recommended. Trichotomy may be useful, and proper care of underwear and bedclothes is necessary to prevent reinfestation.

Suggested Reading

Elston DM (2005) Drugs used in the treatment of pediculosis. J Drugs Dermatol 4:207-11

Ko CJ, Elston DM (2004) Pediculosis. J Am Acad Dermatol 50:1-12

Micali G, Lacarrubba F, Massimino D, Schwartz RA (2011) Dermatoscopy: alternative uses in daily clinical practice. J Am Acad Dermatol 64:1135-46

Scott GR, Chosidow O, IUSTI/WHO (2011) European guideline for the management of pediculosis pubis, 2010. Int J STD AIDS 22:304-5

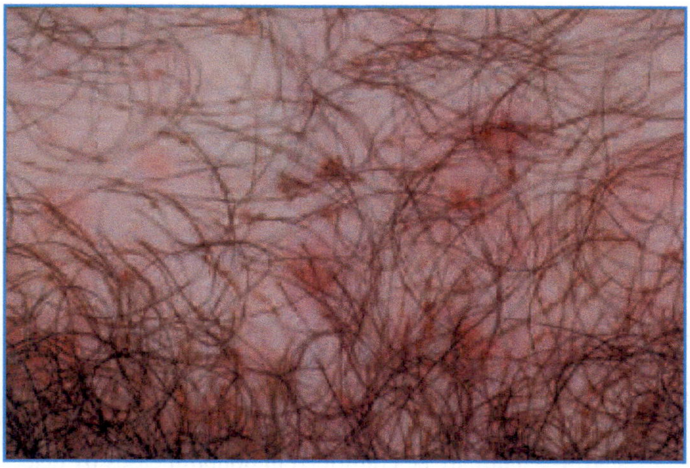

Fig. 3.1 Multiple parasites and nits on the pubis

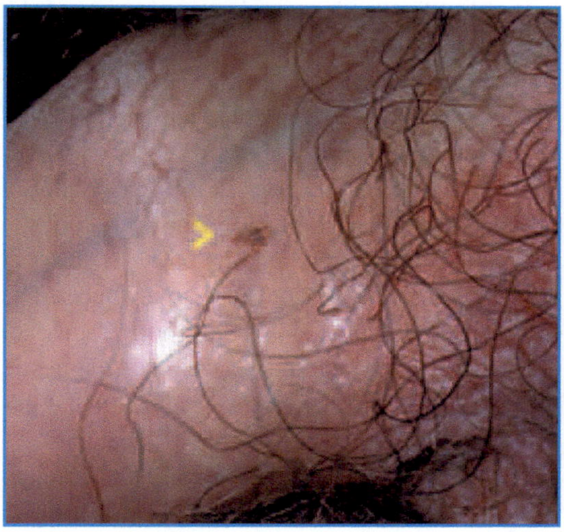

Fig. 3.2 Localization of the parasite on the shaft

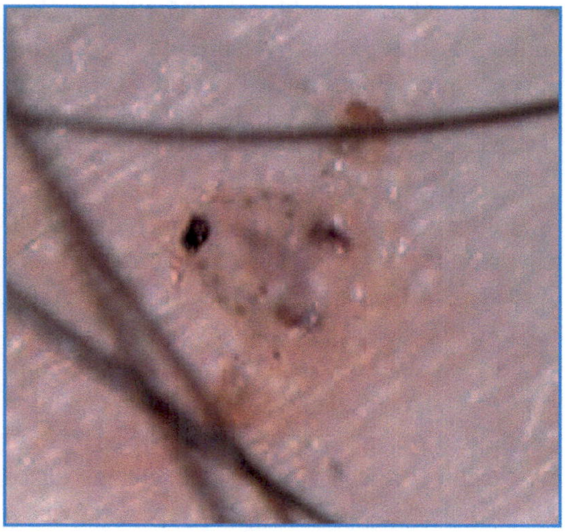

Fig. 3.3 Videodermatoscopy (X80) showing *Phthirus pubis* on the skin

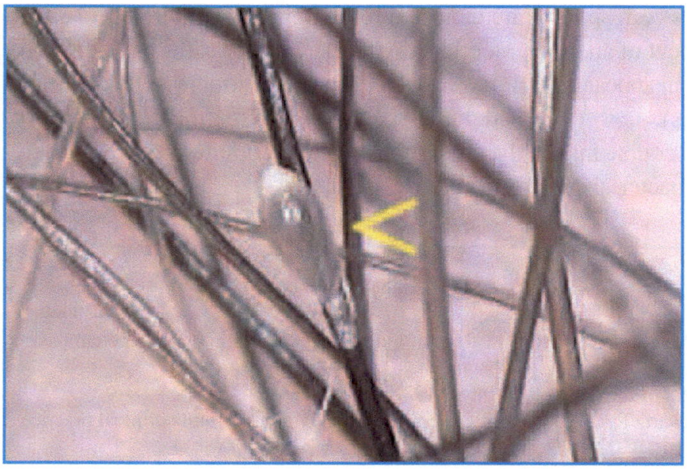

Fig. 3.4 Videodermatoscopy (X80) showing a full, viable nit appearing as an opaque structure, with a rounded free ending, fixed to the pubic hair shaft

Scabies

Definition: scabies is an ectoparasitosis characterized by itching, scratch marks, and presence of multiple burrows that are barely detectable at naked-eye observation.

Etiology: the condition is caused by a mite named *Sarcoptes scabiei hominis*. Pregnant females dig burrows in the stratum corneum, spawning eggs at their end. After 3-4 days new mites come out and reach adulthood in 15-18 days. Contamination may occur by either direct (notably during sexual intercourse) or indirect contact (clothing, bedding). The mite can survive in the environment for 24-36 hours. Scabies is classified as a sexually transmitted disease.

Epidemiology: it is a very common disorder. It has a worldwide spread, and may affect individuals of all ages, races, and socioeconomic classes. About 1-10% of the global population is estimated to be infected with scabies. Genital involvement is common, especially in adult sexually active men.

Clinical appearance: it is characterized by stubborn itching, particularly intense at night, associated with skin markings resulting from repeated scratching. A careful physical examination can reveal the presence of burrows in infestated skin areas, especially on the finger web spaces, flexor wrists, armpits, and periumbilical region. Moreover, in male patients, discrete reddish nodules corresponding to healing lesions with development of an inflammatory granulomatous reaction can appear on the scrotum and penis (nodular scabies).

Clinical course: if not treated, its course may become chronic and complicated by bacterial superinfections. In debilitated or immune suppressed patients the infestation may evolve into a generalized hyperkeratotic and crusty dermatosis, mainly involving the hands and feet, known as Norwegian scabies.

Diagnosis: the clinical diagnosis is usually easy, but may be confirmed in doubtful cases by detection of the mite, and/or its eggs, and/or its excrements, by direct microscopic examination of the scales, obtained from a skin scraping. Videodermatoscopy at low magnification (X10-X40) shows the presence of a small dark brown triangular structure located at the end of the burrow (*jet with contrail*). Higher magnifications (X100-X600) allow a more detailed inspection and identification of the morphology of the mite and its products: its oval translucent body, legs, rostrum, eggs and feces. The exam is not painful, and it is thus more readily accepted than scraping (the traditional diagnostic technique requiring the use of a scalpel blade), especially by children and very nervous patients.

Therapy: permethrin, a topical insecticide, is the treatment of choice. One application is generally effective. For moderate to severe cases another dose may be applied after 7-14 days. Other treatments include benzyl benzoate, crotamiton, malathion and lindane. Antihistamines are indicated for itching and antibiotics for superinfections. After healing, pruritus can persist for a few weeks. Proper treatment of clothes and bedclothes is essential. Treatment must involve the entire household or community to prevent reinfestation.

Suggested Reading

Bongiorno MR, Ferro G, Aricò M (2009) Norwegian (crusted) scabies of glans penis in an immunocompetent patient. Br J Dermatol 161:195-7

Buechner SA (2002) Common skin disorders of the penis. BJU Int 90:498-506

Micali G, Lacarrubba F, Massimino D, Schwartz RA (2011) Dermatoscopy: alternative uses in daily clinical practice. J Am Acad Dermatol 64:1135-46

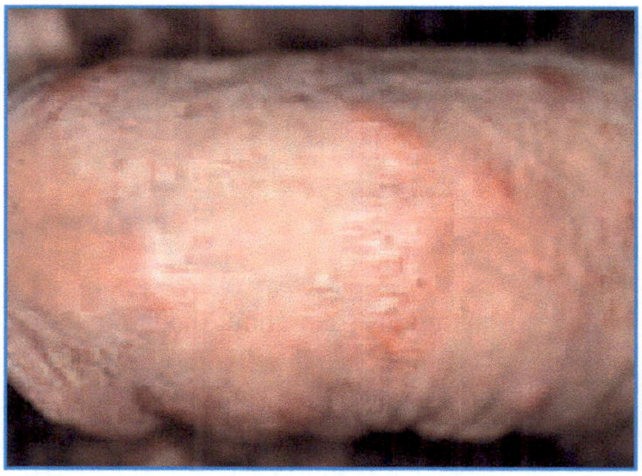

Fig. 3.5 Multiple reddish papules of the shaft

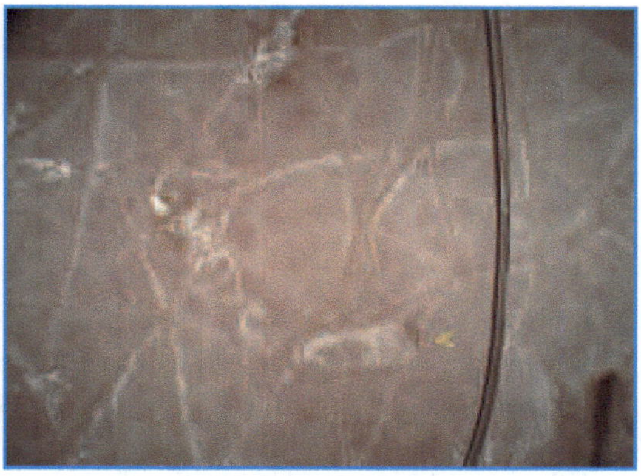

Fig. 3.6 Videodermatoscopy observation (X100) showing the burrow of a mite at its lower end (*arrow*)

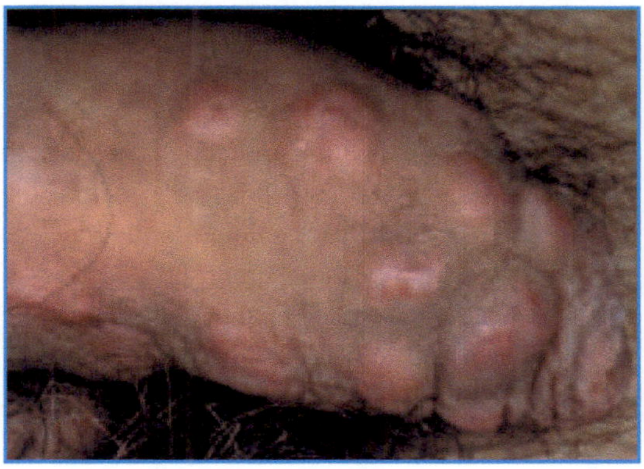

Fig. 3.7 Nodular scabies: multiple nodular lesions on the shaft

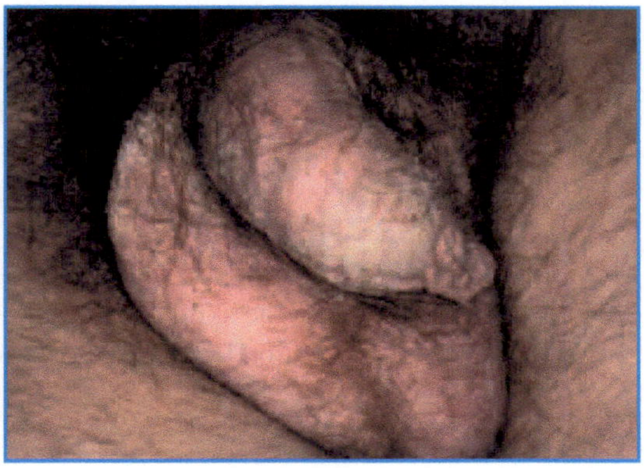

Fig. 3.8 Crusted scabies: confluent and crusted lesions filled with parasites in an HIV+ patient

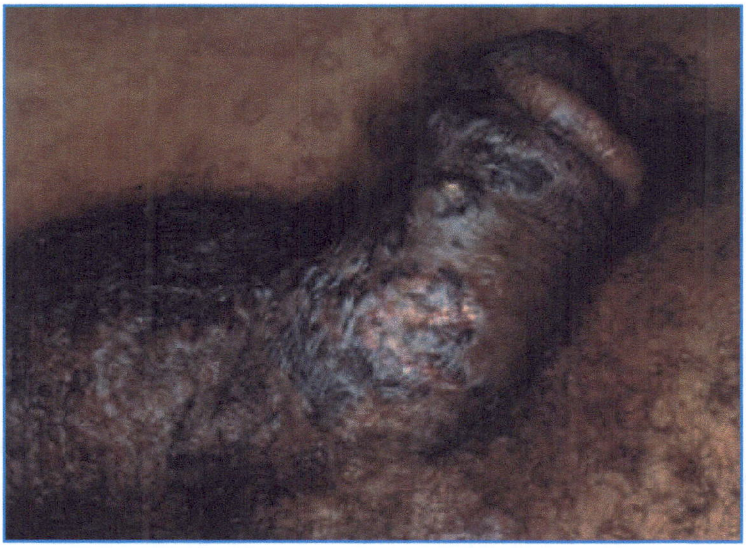

Fig. 3.9 Multiple scratch marks involving the penis and the scrotum in an HIV+ Afro-American patient

Larva Migrans

Definition: Larva Migrans (LM) is a distinctive cutaneous parasitosis characterized by one or more serpiginous lesions. It is commonly known as "creeping eruption".

Etiology: LM is caused by the filariform larva of dog and cat hookworms (*Ancylostoma caninum* and *Ancylostoma brasiliensis*, respectively). Following contact with the contaminated ground of exposed areas, the larva enters the skin through slight epidermal abrasions or through follicles. After penetration, it moves quickly (up to 5 cm a day), excavating a tunnel in the lower epidermal layers and in the upper dermis.

Epidemiology: LM is endemic in tropical and subtropical countries.

Clinical appearance: a small, itchy erythematous papule appears on the skin after penetration of the larva. Its migration leads to the development of a sinuous tract about 0.5-2 mm wide, which may reach a length of some centimetres. This lesion is generally single, but sometimes more than one lesion, arranged in a network pattern, may be found. Itching is always present. The feet and the hands are a common site of involvement. Penile lesions are very unusual and they have rarely been reported.

Clinical course: LM is self-healing but can persist for many months if untreated.

Diagnosis: it is usually easily made based on patient history and from typical clinical features.

Therapy: the lesions can be treated with cryotherapy or with oral albendazole. Albendazole is considered the drug of choice, and systemic therapy is mandatory in case of multiple lesions. In endemic countries avoidance of contact with the contaminated soil of beaches is recommended.

Suggested Reading

Karthikeyan K, Thappa DM, Jeevankumar B (2003) Cutaneous larva migrans of the penis. Sex Transm Infect 79:500

Patel S, Sethi A (2009) Imported tropical diseases. Dermatol Ther 22:538-49

Rao R, Prabhu S, Sripathi H (2007) Cutaneous larva migrans of the genitalia. Indian J Dermatol Venereol Leprol 73:270-1

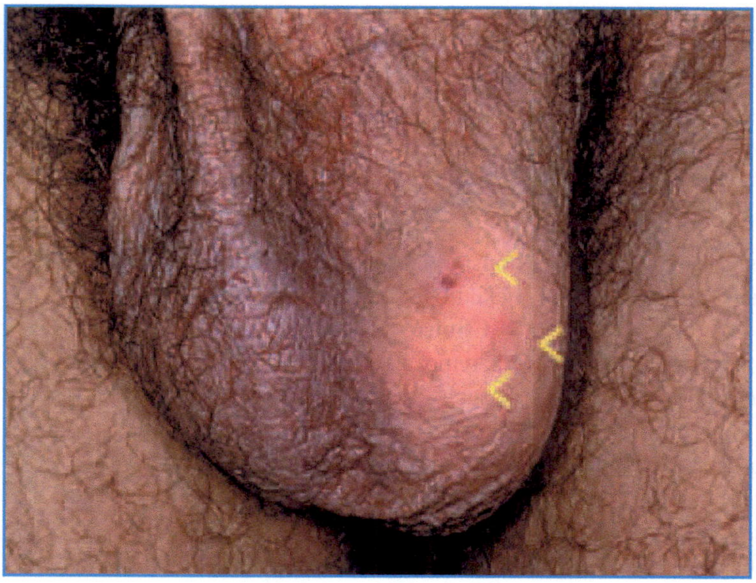

Fig. 3.10 Typical reddish, sinuous, and raised tract on the scrotum

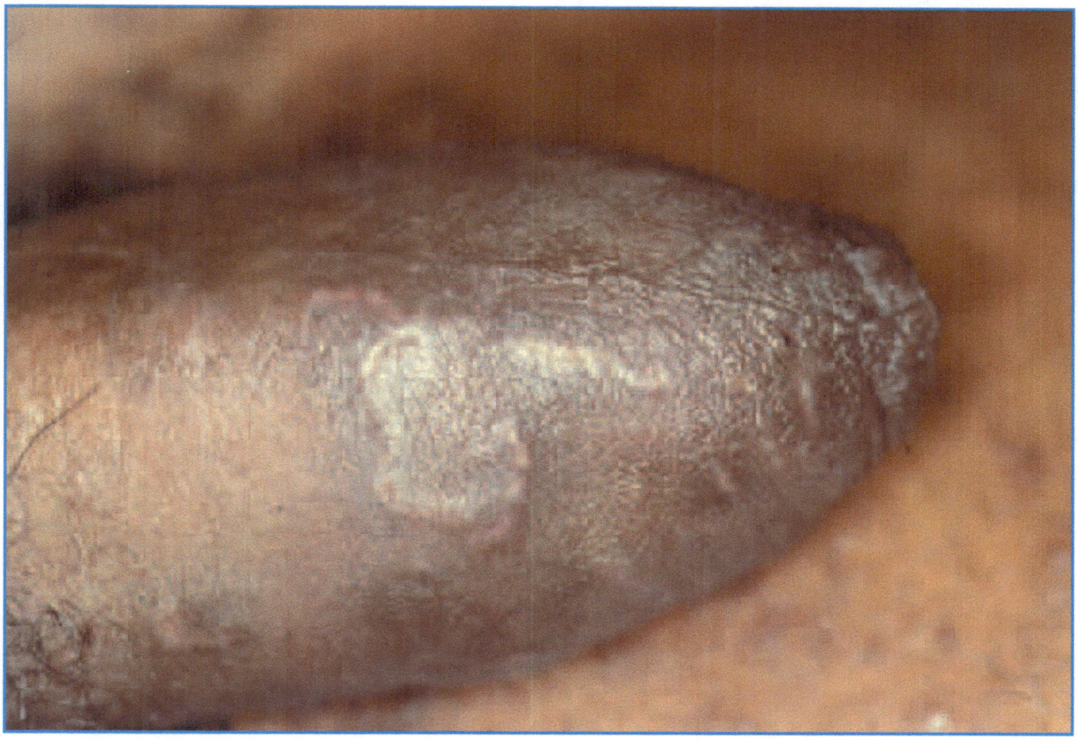

Fig. 3.11 Typical sinuous and raised tract on the shaft in an Afro-American patient

Tick Bites

Definition: they are punctures caused by blood-feeding external parasites which can cause local and systemic complications.

Etiology: different types of ticks exist, some of which are able to bite humans. They are often harmless, but sometimes they may carry troublesome systemic infectious disorders. Ticks of the genus Ixodes (*I. ricinus*) are the main vectors of Lyme disease; *Riphicephalus sanguineus* is implicated in the genesis of rickettiosis.

Epidemiology: tick infestations are more frequent in spring.

Clinical appearance: they mostly affect covered skin areas, where the ticks attach to maintain their blood meal. Secondary bacterial skin infection, allergic reactions, and granuloma formation may ensue. Finally, some diseases potentially transmitted by a tick bite include Lyme disease, rickettiosis, and virus encephalitis.

Clinical course: it is often uneventful after tick removal, unless infective complications occur. In such cases, the diseases follow their natural history. Tick paralysis is a relatively rare complication but it can be fatal.

Diagnosis: ticks are readily identified by clinical observation.

Therapy: apart from the general rules for tick bite prevention, any tick found should be immediately and completely removed alive. Furthermore, the technique used to remove the tick should not allow or cause infective body fluids to escape through the tick into the wound site. Any local or systemic complication should be sought out and properly treated.

Suggested Reading

Hynote ED, Mervine PC, Stricker RB (2012) Clinical evidence for rapid transmission of Lyme disease following a tick-bite. Diagn Microbiol Infect Dis 72:188-92

Roupakias S, Mitsakou P, Nimer AA (2011) Tick removal. J Prev Med Hyg 52:40-4

Tappe D, Dobler G, Stich A (2009) Tache noire in African tick bite fever. Am J Trop Med Hyg 81:733-4

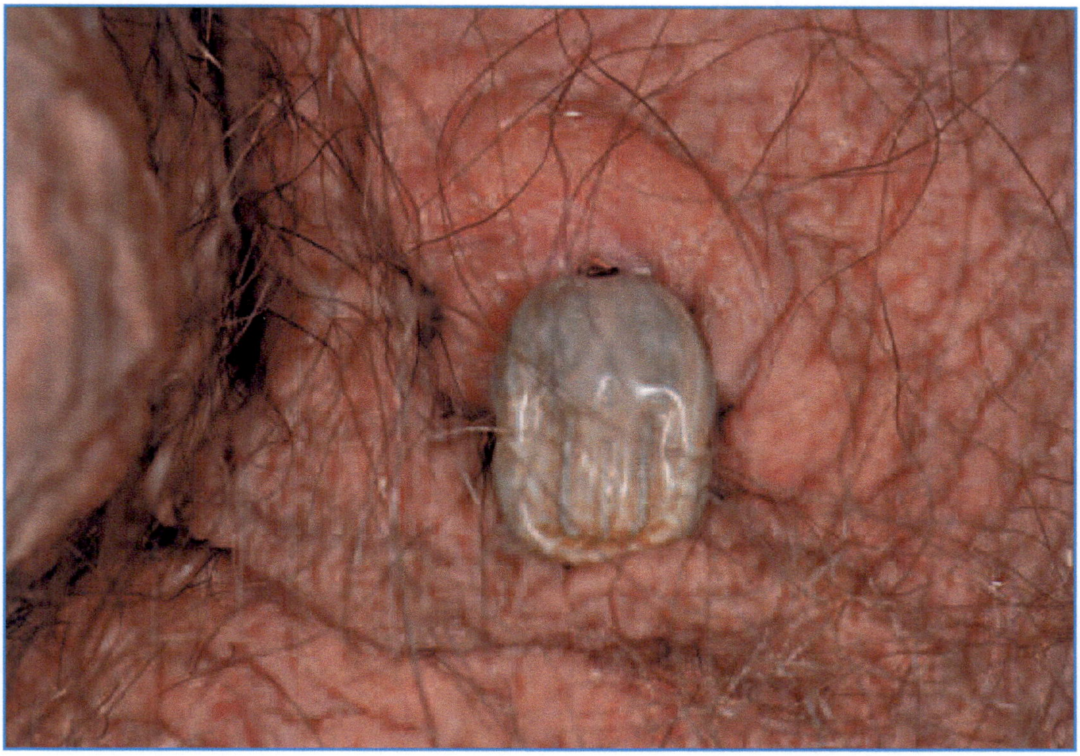

Fig. 3.12 Localization of the parasite on the scrotum

4 Sexually Transmitted Diseases

Franco Dinotta, Stefano Ramoni, Pompeo Donofrio, and Marco Cusini

F. Dinotta (✉)
Center for Sexually Transmitted Diseases
Dermatology Unit
Dipartimento di Specialità Medico-Chirurgiche
AOU "Policlinico – Vittorio Emanuele"
Presidio "G. Rodolico", Catania, Italy
e-mail: f.dinotta@unict.it

G. Micali et al., *Atlas of Male Genital Disorders*,
DOI: 10.1007/978-88-470-2787-9_4, © Springer-Verlag Italia 2013

Syphilis

Definition: syphilis is a transmittable bacterial disease that predominantly affects the genital area. It is characterized by different clinical stages alternating with long asymptomatic periods.

Etiology: it is a sexually transmitted disease caused by *Treponema Pallidum* (TP) *sub species pallidum*, a gram-negative bacterium. Approximately 30% of those exposed become infected.

Epidemiology: syphilis has a worldwide spread, and in recent years its incidence has been rising in the western world. This increase has been particularly striking in metropolitan areas and among homosexual men. The disease is more common in males, but its real frequency may be underestimated in women because female genital primary lesions are often unnoticed.

Clinical appearance: primary syphilis is characterized by a solitary, reddish, indurated, often eroded and painless nodule localized at the site of TP inoculation. This chancre usually occurs in the genital area, but it has been described on almost any site of the body. Coexistent regional lymphadenopathy, usually healing in about 1 month, is typical.

The clinical manifestations of secondary syphilis include polymorphic cutaneous eruptions, mucous lesions, diffused lymphadenopathy, and systemic symptoms. The most frequent cutaneous findings include roseola syphilitica and papular syphilis. The former consists of a large number of round or oval erythematous patches, a few millimiters in diameter, symmetrically distributed on both sides of the trunk and upper limbs. Papular syphilis is characterized by an eruption of erythematous or reddish-brown papules, sometimes covered by scales, widely distributed on the skin and frequently involving the palms and soles. Mucosal lesions occurring at this stage include soft, flat vegetations involving the genital and perigenital area.

The third stage of the disease can affect any organ, but it is mainly characterized by neurological involvement. The cutaneous manifestations of tertiary syphilis include nodular syphilis, characterized by painless, indurated, dull red nodules of varying size that may occur on any part of the body, and gummatous syphilis, characterized by deep granulomatous lesions evolving into chronic ulcerations.

Clinical course: TP usually enters the skin during sexual contact, as transmission is facilitated by mucosal or skin erosions that may occur during intercourse. After an incubation period of 20-40 days the primary lesion develops at the portal of entry. The primary chancre, if untreated, lasts for 2-4 weeks and heals spontaneously, normally without scarring. After few weeks, or even

Suggested Reading

Cheng S, French P (2008) Unilateral penile swelling: an unusual presentation of primary syphilis? Int J STD AIDS 19:640-1

Coutinho B, Baranowski U, Miller E (2008) Male patient with a genital ulceration. Primary syphilis. Am Fam Physician 77:215-6

Dinotta F, De Pasquale R, Micali G (2009) Secondary syphilis with exclusive peno-scrotal localization. G Ital Dermatol Venereol 144:725-8

Zou H, Fairley CK, Guy R, Chen MY (2012) The efficacy of clinic-based interventions aimed at increasing screening for bacterial sexually transmitted infections among men who have sex with men: a systematic review. Sex Transm Dis 39:382-7

during healing of the primary chancre, the secondary stage begins. This phase is characterized by relapsing cutaneous rashes, with damage of skin appendages and internal organs. After a period of latency ranging from 3 months to 3 years, tertiary lesions can develop in the internal organs, the central nervous system, and the skin.

Diagnosis: syphilis can be diagnosed by direct and indirect techniques. Direct techniques include dark-field microscopy examination and PCR, both useful for TP detection in the oozing lesions of primary and secondary syphilis. PCR is particularly suitable for extragenital locations, as it can also be performed on skin specimens. Indirect techniques include treponemal (TPHA, TPPA, EIA-Tp, chemiluminescence immune assay) and non-treponemal (VDRL, RPR) serological tests, both useful in identifying the antibody response to the infection. Histology may be helpful for diagnosis in atypical cases only.

Therapy: the first line treatment is systemic penicillin, used at variable dosages depending on the disease stage. In case of penicillin allergy, erythromicin or doxycicline may be used.

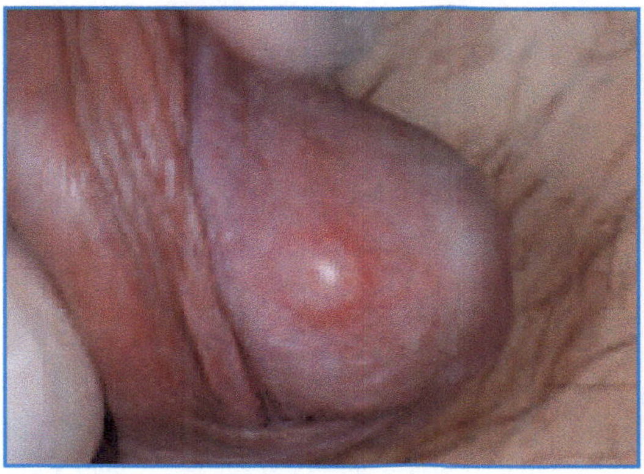

Fig. 4.1 Primary syphilis: reddish and ulcerated nodule on the glans

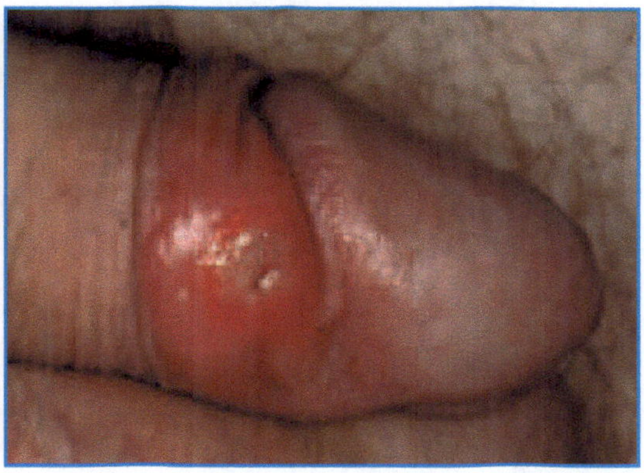

Fig. 4.2 Primary syphilis: typical solitary, reddish, and ulcerated nodule on the coronal sulcus

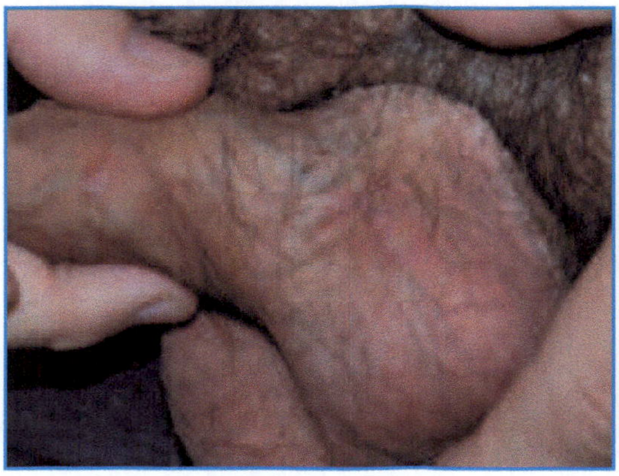

Fig. 4.3 Primary syphilis: multiple and ulcerated nodules on the shaft and scrotum

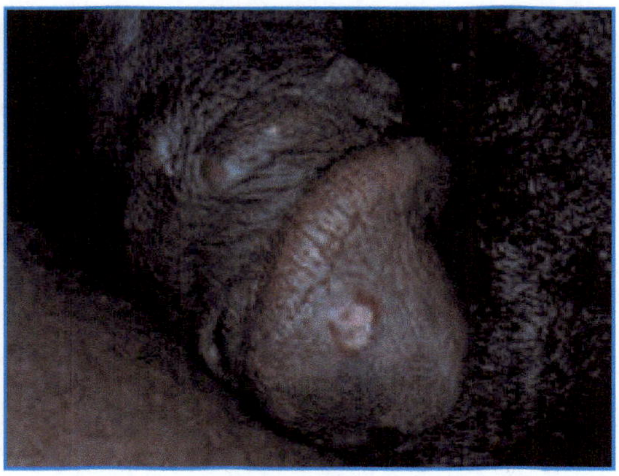

Fig. 4.4 Primary syphilis: multiple ulcerated nodules involving the glans and the shaft in an Afro-American patient

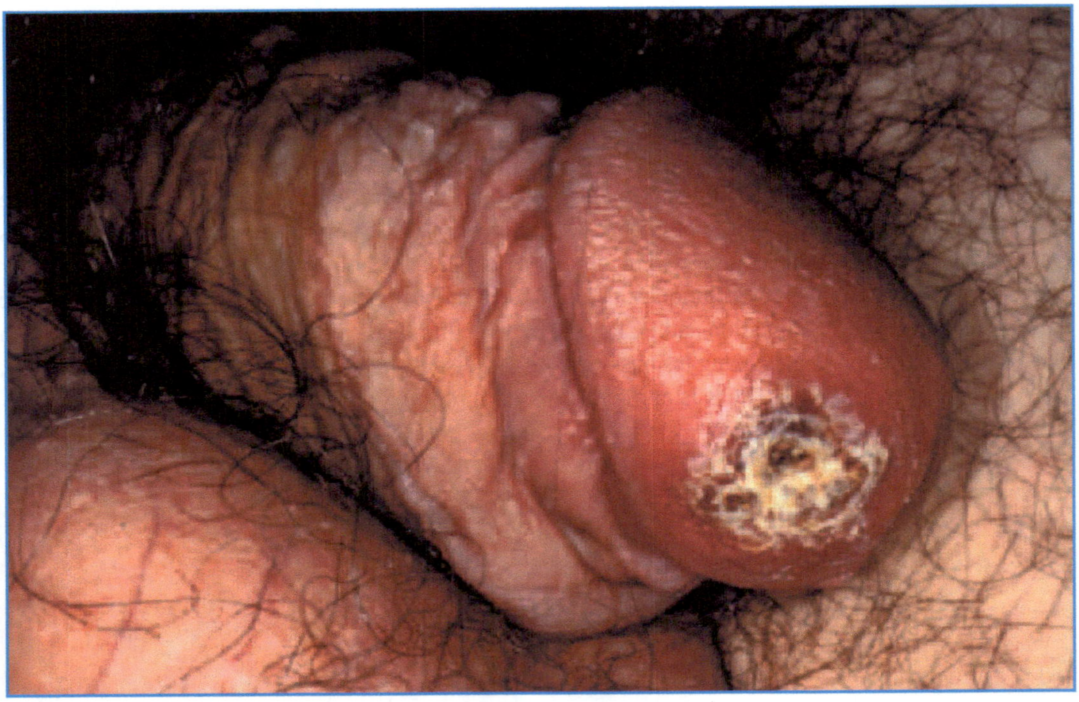

Fig. 4.5 Primary syphilis: nodule on the glans with atypical psoriasiform presentation

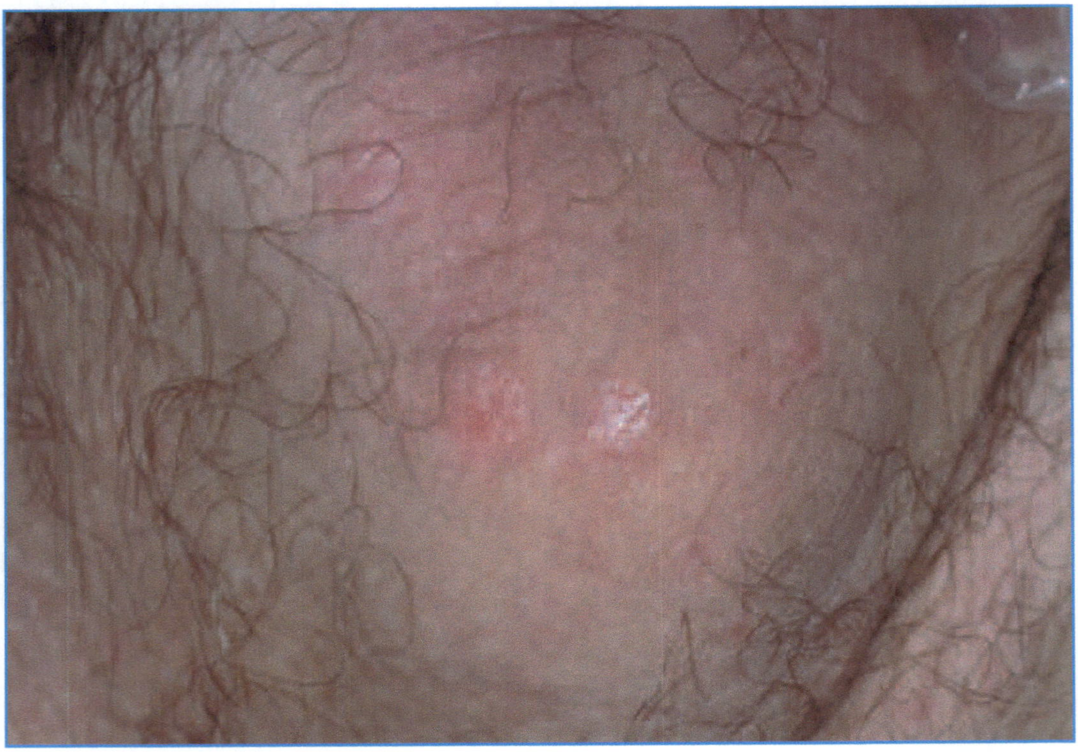

Fig. 4.6 Secondary syphilis: erosions and flat vegetations involving the scrotum and the glans

Granuloma Inguinale

Definition: granuloma inguinale, also called donovanosis, is a chronic bacterial infection with frequent relapses, affecting the genital area.

Etiology: it is a sexually transmitted disease caused by *Klebsiella granulomatosis* and *Calymmatobacterium granulomatis*, a rod-shaped gram-negative agent formerly called *Donovania granulomatis*. This microrganism has an incubation period ranging from 8 days to 12 weeks, with an average of 2 to 4 weeks.

Epidemiology: it is a very rare disease in Europe and North America. Donovanosis is endemic in tropical or subtropical countries, where it is associated with poverty and poor hygiene. In tropical countries, about 20% of male patients with sexually transmitted diseases have granuloma inguinale. Peak incidence occurs between the ages of 20-40 years; men are more infected than women. There are approximately 100 cases/yr reported in the United States.

Clinical appearance: in early stages, asymptomatic papules and nodes develop in the genital or perigenital area. Subsequently, lesions evolve into painless, foul-smelling ulcerations surrounded by a peripheral inflammatory reaction, which bleed easily if traumatized. As the ulcers slowly expand centrifugally and become granulomatous, patients develop subcutaneous granulomas in the inguinal regions, usually without lymph node involvement. Extragenital lesions, notably involving the oral cavity, have been reported. Abdominal visceral dissemination has been observed, mostly in endemic regions. In such instances, systemic symptoms, such as fever, malaise, anemia, and weight loss, usually occur.

Clinical course: the disease has a slow and gradual onset, beginning with an inconspicuous pimple or lumpy eruption on the skin. If untreated, the ulcerative lesions persist, with possible superinfection by other sexually transmitted agents, leading to mutilation and destruction of the genital tissue. In addition, the scar tissue produced by late stage infection may cause urethral stenosis. Local lymphatic damage may lead, less commonly in men than in women, to chronic edema and elephantiasis. A high risk of genital cancer has also been reported.

Diagnosis: the diagnosis of granuloma inguinale is made by tissue smears or biopsy or both. The demonstration of intracytoplasmic bacteria (Donovan bodies) in mononuclear cells confirms the diagnosis. More recently, PCR methods have been developed.

Therapy: granuloma inguinale is treated with oral antibiotics administered for at least 3 weeks. The use of azythromicin and doxycycline is recommended. Alternative treatments include tetracycline, trimethoprim-sulfamethoxazol, erythromycin, and ciprofloxacin. Although the skin ulcers will start to show signs of healing in about a week, the patient must take the full course of medication to minimize the possibility of relapse.

Suggested Reading

Bezerra SM, Jardim MM, Silva VB (2011) Granuloma inguinale (Donovanosis). An Bras Dermatol 86:585-6

O'Farrell N, Moi H, IUSTI/WHO European STD guidelines Editorial Board (2010) European guideline for the management of donovanosis, 2010. Int J STD AIDS 21:609-10

Roett MA, Mayor MT, Uduhiri KA (2012) Diagnosis and management of genital ulcers. Am Fam Physician 85:254-62

Velho PE, Souza EM, Belda Junior W (2008) Donovanosis. Braz J Infect Dis 12:521-5

Lymphogranuloma Venereum

Definition: Lymphogranuloma Venereum (LV), also known as Durand-Nicolas-Favre disease, is a bacterial infection of the lymphatic system characterized by acute inguinal lymphadenitis and genital ulceration.

Etiology: the etiological agent of LV is *Chlamydia trachomatis*, serotypes L1, L2, L3. It is a sexually transmitted disease. Its incubation period ranges from 3 to 30 days.

Epidemiology: LV is widespread in tropical and subtropical areas of Africa and Asia. It is more frequent in men.

Clinical appearance: the initial lesion is often a papule or shallow ulcer in the groin area. A painless sore or lump may be visible in correspondence to the bacteria portal of entry. Because the sore or lump is usually painless and clears up without treatment, it often goes unnoticed. During the second stage, groin lymph nodes may become swollen on one or both sides. Perirectal lymph nodes may also be affected as a result of anal intercourse. When inguinal and femoral nodes are enlarged, they are characteristically separated by Poupart's ligament (sign of Greenblatt). Fever, malaise, headache and arthralgias may sometimes be present. Physical examination may also show drainage of groin lymph nodes through the skin. Diarrhea and lower abdominal pain may ensue.

Clinical course: the primary genital lesion is usually transient and painless. After it heals, lymphadenitis occurs, followed by the genitoanorectal syndrome. Lymphadenitis is usually unilateral and affects multiple inguinal nodes. Untreated, LV persists for several months or years. Possible complications include elephantiasis, anal stenosis, and rectal strictures.

Diagnosis: it is essentially clinical, and it is confirmed by the LV complement fixation test (LV-CFT) and by laboratory tests devised for Chlamydiae detection. Culture of *C. trachomatis*, although useful for definitive diagnostic confirmation, is technically costly and time-consuming. The best results are obtained using aspirates from an involved inguinal lymph node. Other tests for LV include microimmunofluorescence and polymerase chain reaction. Further tests to rule out other sexually transmitted infections that might have been transmitted at the same time are strongly recommended.

Therapy: oral antibiotics are indicated. The treatment of choice is doxycycline, although tetracycline, erythromycin, and azithromycin are also effective. Incision and surgical drainage of the purulent discharge above the inguinal ligament may minimize symptoms.

Suggested Reading

Cusini M, Boneschi V, Arancio L et al (2009) Lymphogranuloma venereum: the italian experience. Sex Trans Infect 85:171-2

Greene L, Rubinstein L, Gaffney J et al (2008) Lymphogranuloma venereum in the UK in 2003. Int J STD AIDS 19:139-40

Kapoor S (2008) Re-emergence of lymphogranuloma venereum. J Eur Acad Dermatol Venereol 22:409-16

Roett MA, Mayor MT, Uduhiri KA (2012) Diagnosis and management of genital ulcers. Am Fam Physician 85:254-62

Vargas-Leguas H, Garcia de Olalla P, Arando M et al (2012) Lymphogranuloma venereum: a hidden emerging problem, Barcelona, 2011. Euro Surveill 17

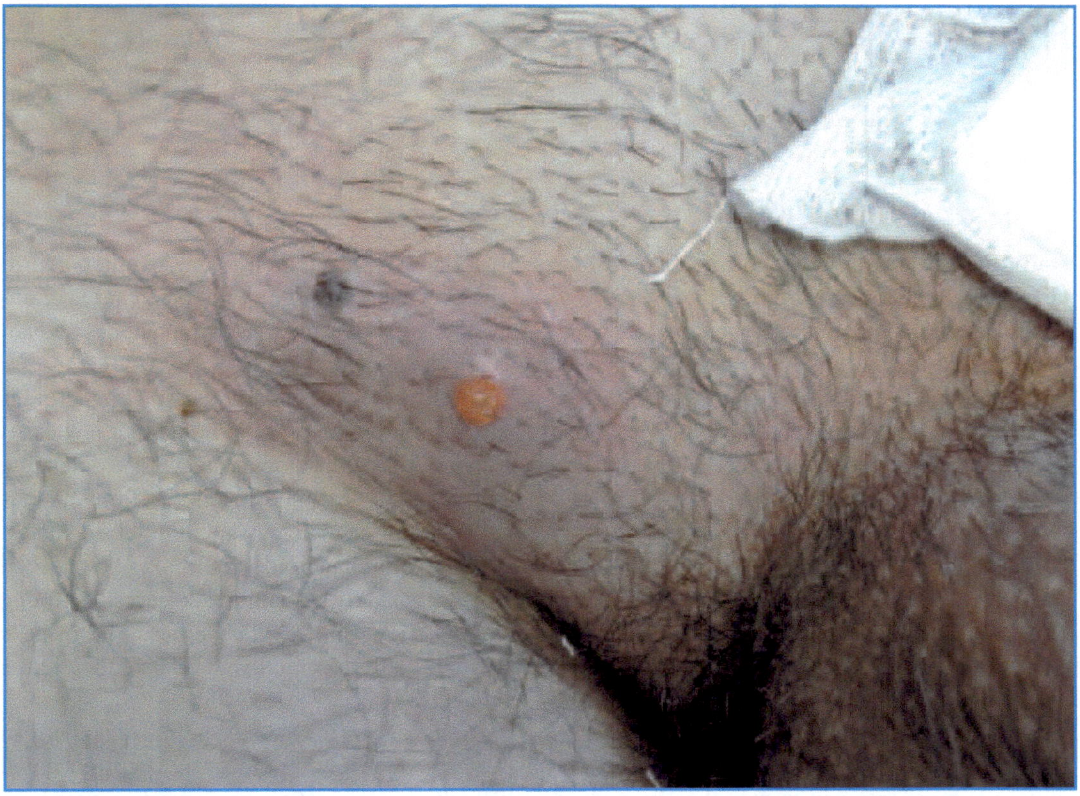

Fig. 4.7 Unilateral inguinal lymphadenitis with evidence of drainage

Chancroid

Definition: chancroid is a highly contagious bacterial infection characterized by the presence of painful ulcers and inflammatory inguinal adenopathy in the groin area.

Etiology: it is caused by *Haemophilus ducreyi*, a small gram-negative streptobacillus transmitted during sexual intercourse. In men the incubation period ranges from 5 to 14 days.

Epidemiology: chancroid is very common in Africa and it is becoming more common in other countries. Its real incidence is difficult to determine and probably underestimated, due to the unavailablity of diagnostic resources in underdeveloped countries where the disease is prevalent, and because of the difficulties in culturing *H. ducreyi* even when laboratory facilities are available. The disease is more frequent in men than in women. Uncircumcised men seem to be at higher risk than circumcised ones.

Clinical appearance: it usually begins as a small papule that rapidly becomes pustular and erodes, leading to the development of a painful ulcer 1 to 2 cm in diameter with sharply defined, undermined irregular borders. The ulcerations, soft and covered by a grayish material, can be single or multiple, but in the majority of cases two clustered lesions of variable size (5-50 mm) may develop. They are very painful and bleed easily, and in men they are generally localized on the penis. Lymphadenopathy is usually unilateral, and in 50% of cases the lymph nodal swelling is followed by a break in the skin which causes draining abscesses. The enlarged lymph nodes and abscesses are called buboes.

Clinical course: without therapy, chancroid is self-healing in about 1-2 months. In a few cases it can persist for some years with a relapsing course. Complications include urethral fistulas and foreskin scarring in uncircumcised males. Patients with chancroid should also be checked for other sexually transmitted diseases, including syphilis, HIV, and genital herpes. The disease does not confer immunity, so that reinfection is frequent.

Diagnosis: it may easily be misdiagnosed in Western countries due to its rare occurrence and difficulties in detecting the causative pathogen (*H. ducreyi* is difficult to cultivate). Diagnosis is made by the demonstration of *H. ducreyi* in the ulcerative lesions using microbial cultures or nucleic acid amplification techniques. In doubtful cases, histopathological examination can be useful.

Therapy: antibiotic treatment with azithromycin, ceftriaxone or erythromycin cures the infection, resolves symptoms and prevents transmission to others. Large lymph node swellings need to be drained, either with a needle or local surgery. If treatment is successful, ulcers usually improve in about a week. The time required for complete healing is generally related to the size of the ulcer.

Suggested Reading

Bhunu CP, Mushayabasa S (2011) Chancroid transmission dynamics: a mathematical modeling approach. Theory Biosci 130:289-98

Hope-Rapp E, Anyfantakis V, Fouéré S et al (2010) Etiology of genital ulcer disease. A prospective study of 278 cases seen in an STD clinic in Paris. Sex Transm Dis 37:153-8

Kemp M, Christensen JJ, Lautenschlager S et al (2011) European guideline for the management of chancroid, 2011. Int J STD AIDS 22:241-4

Li W, Janowicz DM, Fortney KR et al (2009) Mechanism of human natural killer cell activation by Haemophilus ducreyi. J Infect Dis 200:590-8

Roett MA, Mayor MT, Uduhiri KA (2012) Diagnosis and management of genital ulcers. Am Fam Physician 85:254-62

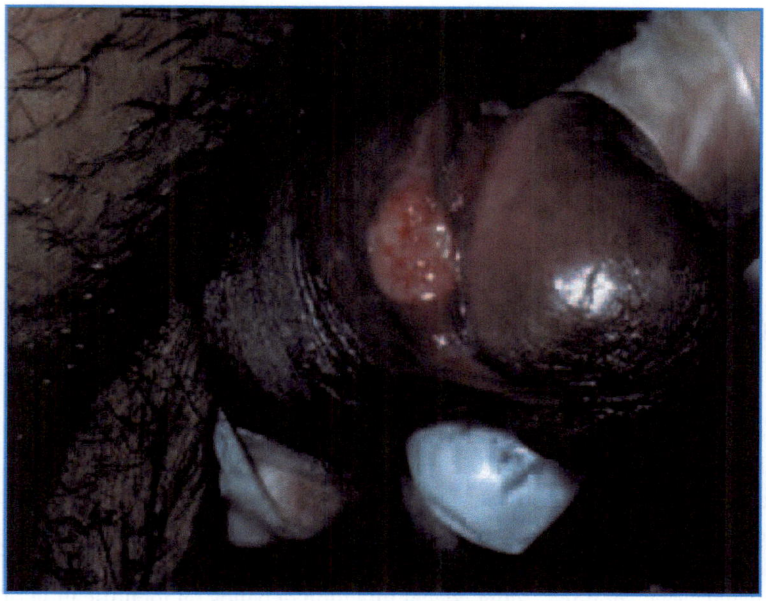

Fig. 4.8 Sharply defined ulcer, covered by a grayish material, of the foreskin in an Afro-American patient

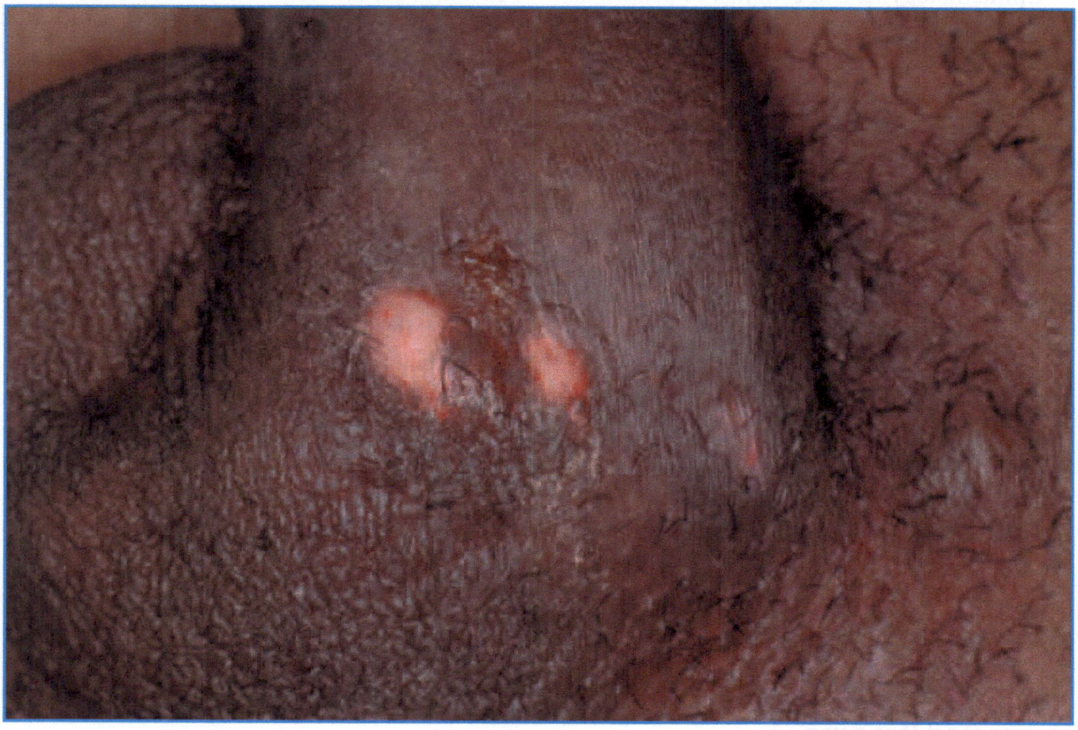

Fig. 4.9 Multiple ulcers located on the proximal shaft

Gonorrhea

Definition: gonorrhea is a bacterial infection characterized by acute inflammation at the site of inoculation, with possible local and systemic complications.

Etiology: the etiological agent is *Neisseria gonorrhoeae* (a small gram-negative diplococcus). It infects predominantly the noncornified epithelium of the urogenital tract, rectum, oropharynx and conjunctivae. Gonorrhea is generally transmitted by sexual contact or perinatally. Indirect transmission is very unusual as *N. gonorrhoeae* dies rapidly in the outside environment. The incubation period is 2-7 days.

Epidemiology: it is a common infectious disease, affecting both sexes with a higher prevalence in males. The highest incidence of gonorrhea is in young adults (15-29 years). Incidence has fallen substantially in the last decade, perhaps due to gonorrhea control programs. It is the cause of approximately 1/3 of all urethritis in the United States.

Clinical appearance: the most common presentation of gonorrhea is acute anterior urethritis, with mucopurulent urethral discharge and dysuria. Burning and pain on urination are also present. A few days later, the discharge usually becomes more profuse and, at times, blood-tinged. Acute epididymitis may also occur. Rectal and pharyngeal infections are possible, usually paucisymptomatic or completely asymptomatic.

Clinical course: it most often remains localized to the inoculation site, but, if untreated, it can involve the upper urogenital tract in males, causing complications such as urethral stricture, prostatytis, epididymitis, and cowperitis. A systemic involvement is possible but it is very rare. Disseminated gonococcal infections (bacteremia) occur in about 1-3% of cases, with fever, arthralgia, acute arthritis and tenosynovitis. Typically, these patients often do not report urogenital or pharyngeal complaints.

Diagnosis: traditionally, laboratory diagnosis of gonococcal infection depends on identification of *N. gonorrhoeae* at an infected site with Gram stain and microbial culture. The presence of typical Gram-negative intracellular diplococcic after Gram stain establishes the diagnosis. Isolation through culture is the standard diagnostic clue, and should be used whenever practical. It should be performed if symptoms persist following treatment. However, newer polymerase chain reaction-based testing methods are becoming more common. All those testing positive for gonorrhea should be tested for other sexually transmitted diseases.

Therapy: gonorrhea is effectively treated with penicillin. Because of increasing rates of antibiotic resistance, this issue needs to be taken into account when deciding on treatment. In the UK, the Health Protection Agency has recommended the use of a combination of a single dose of oral azithromycin and intramuscular ceftriaxone as alternative treatment, since injectable ceftriaxone appears to be one of the few effective antibiotics.

Suggested Reading

Bignell C, Fitzgerald M, Guideline Development Group British Association for Sexual Health and HIV UK (2011) UK national guideline for the management of gonorrhoea in adults, 2011. Int J STD AIDS 22:541-7

Bignell C, Ison CA, Jungmann E (2006) Gonorrhoea. Sex Transm Infect 82(Suppl 4):6-9

Newman LM, Moran JS, Workowski KA (2007) Update on the management of gonorrhea in adults in the United States. Clin Infect Dis 44(Suppl 3):S84-101

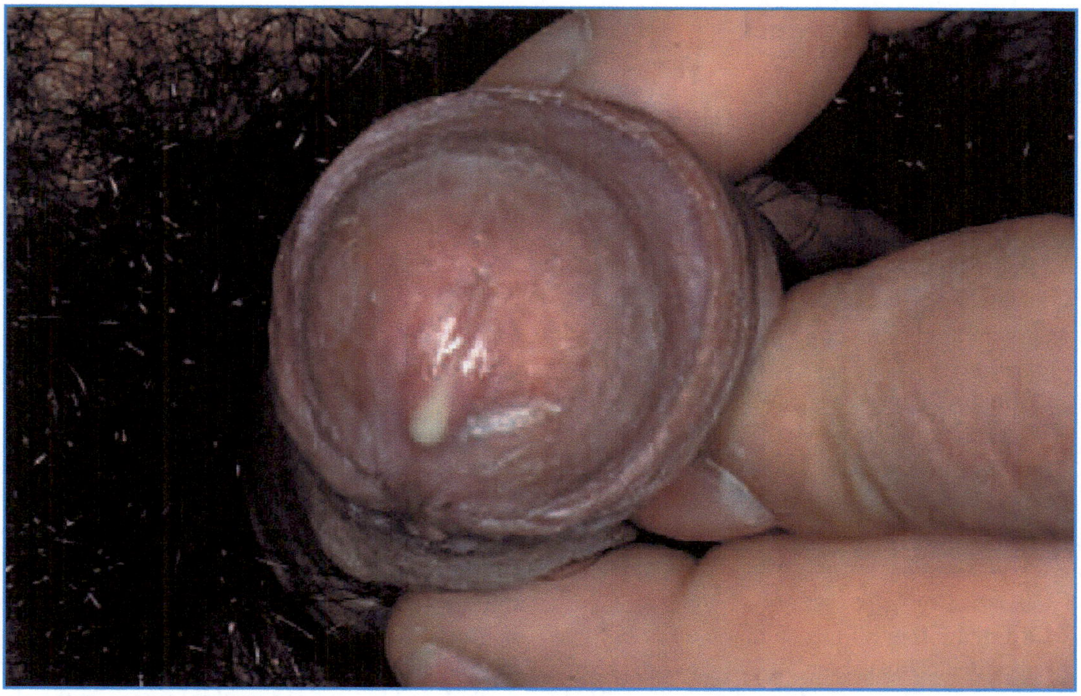

Fig. 4.10 Typical urethritis characterized by mucopurulent discharge

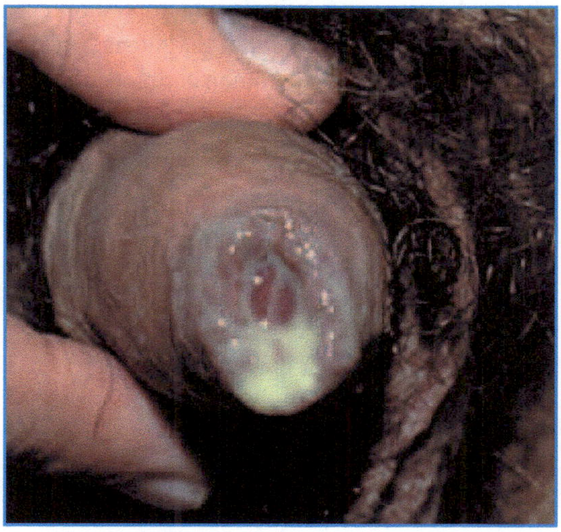

Fig. 4.11 Urethritis with marked mucopurulent discharge

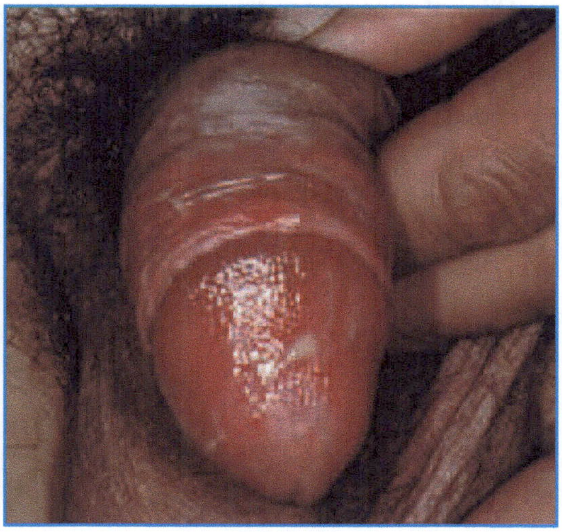

Fig. 4.12 Balanitis characterized by marked erythema and discharge

Nongonococcal Urethritis

Definition: Nongonococcal Urethritis (NGU) is an infectious disease characterized by discharge and/or urethral symptoms not caused by *Neisseria gonorrhoeae*.

Etiology: it may be caused by different organisms, although the most frequent causes are *Chlamydia trachomatis* (subtypes from D to K) and *Mycoplasma genitalium*. Other agents include *Ureaplasma urealyticum*, *Haemophilus vaginalis*, Herpes simplex virus, Adenovirus and *Trichomonas vaginalis*.

Epidemiology: it is a common disease; it has been estimated that about 50% of cases of urethritis are nongonococcal. According to the World Health Organization data, every year 92,000,000 cases of chlamydial infections are registered worldwide, and chlamydial infection is considered one of the most important causes of sterility.

Clinical appearance: the signs and symptoms of NGU are urethral discharge, burning or pain during micturition, itching, irritation or tenderness, and stained underwear. A history of genital infection in the sexual partner is often reported.

Clinical course: if untreated, the disease can spread along the genitourinary tract leading to complications such as prostatitis in men and inflammatory pelvic disease in women. Moreover, irreversible complications such as sterility due to fibrotic evolution can be observed.

Diagnosis: all patients who have confirmed or suspected urethritis should be tested for *N. gonorrhoeae* and *Chlamydiae*. A microscopic and/or culture test of the discharge or of a urine sample can reveal the infection. Microscopic examination is mandatory for differential diagnosis with gonorrhea. In NGU it reveals more than 5 polymorphonuclear leukocytes (x1000) in a Gram- or methylene blue-stained urethral smear, in the absence of *Neisseria* identification. The most reliable method to differentiate chlamydial from mycoplasma infections is the use of nucleic acid amplification techniques. Urethritis due to mechanical injury and irritating factors should be considered in the differential diagnosis.

Therapy: the most common antibiotics used to treat NGU are doxycycline or azithromycin. NGU from *T. vaginalis* should be treated with metronidazole or tinidazole plus azithromycin.

Suggested Reading

Azariah S, Reid M (2000) Adenovirus and non-gonococcal urethritis. Int J STD AIDS 11:548-50

Seña A, Lensing S, Rompalo A et al (2012) Chlamydia trachomatis, Mycoplasma genitalium, and Trichomonas vaginalis infections in men with non-gonococcal urethritis: predictors and persistence after therapy. J Infect Dis 206:357-65

Shahmanesh M, Moi H, Lassau F, Janier M, IUSTI/WHO (2009) 2009 European guideline on the management of male non-gonococcal urethritis. Int J STD AIDS 20:458-64

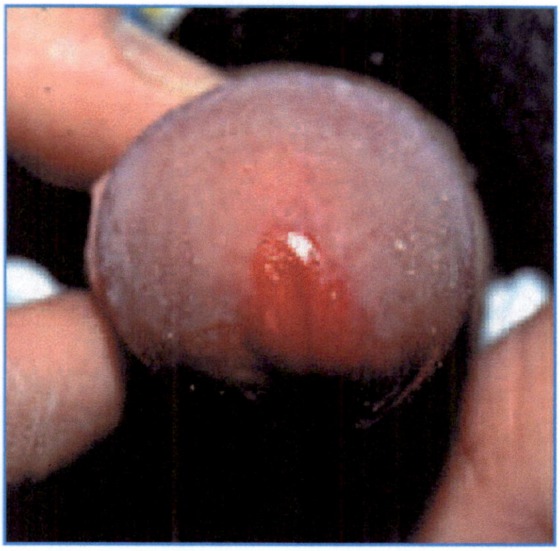

Fig. 4.13 Erythema of the meatus

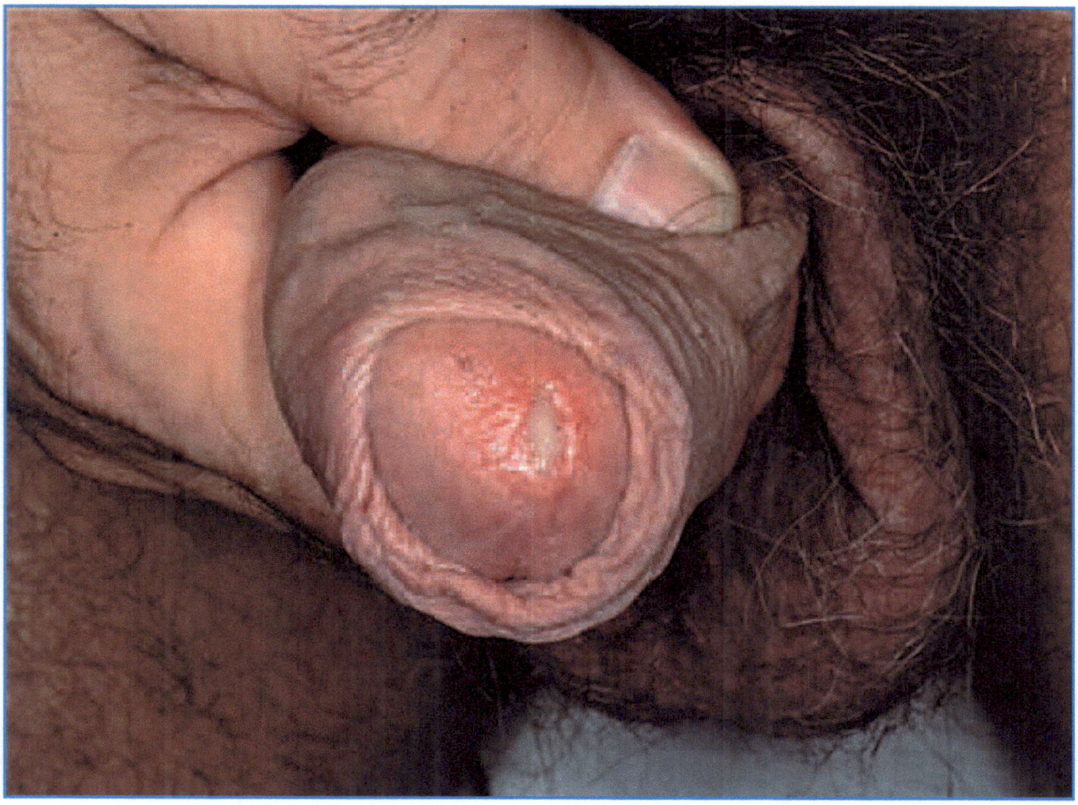

Fig. 4.14 Evidence of urethral discharge

5 Inflammatory Disorders

Maria Rita Nasca, Francesco Lacarrubba, Maria Letizia Musumeci, and Giuseppe Micali

M.R. Nasca (✉)
Dermatology Unit
AOU "Policlinico – Vittorio Emanuele"
Presidio "G. Rodolico", Catania, Italy
e-mail: nasca@policlinico.unict.it

G. Micali et al., *Atlas of Male Genital Disorders*,
DOI: 10.1007/978-88-470-2787-9_5, © Springer-Verlag Italia 2013

Contact Dermatitis (Irritant/Allergic)

Definition: contact dermatitis is an inflammation of the skin caused by contact with certain substances. Based on pathogenesis, two distinct types of contact dermatitis may be identified: Irritant Contact Dermatitis (ICD) and Allergic Contact Dermatitis (ACD).

Etiology: ICD is a nonimmunologic inflammatory response induced by exposure to chemical agents (alkali, hydrofluoric acid, solvents) or urine and feces in incontinent patients, directly damaging the skin, while ACD is a delayed type IV sensitivity (allergy) to specific sensitizing agents (allergens) that come into contact with the skin. The commonest allergens in genital areas include topical medications, additives in personal hygiene products, condoms, and piercing. Saliva and semen can rarely be allergenic.

Epidemiology: both ICD and ACD may occur at any age and are more frequent in women than men (female-to-male ratio 2:1). Both forms have a prevalence of about 4 cases per 10,000 individuals. They are more common during adulthood, and they are thought to be more prevalent among whites.

Clinical appearance: in the acute stage, erythema, edema, and possible blistering with exudation are present. Chronic lesions are usually dry, thickened, fissured, and scaly. In the moist genital area, scaling is often less noticeable. ACD is characterized by pruritic papules and vesicles on an erythematous base. ICD can show different patterns, with macular erythema, edema or vesiculation. Chronic ICD may have hyperkeratosis and ACD lichenification. Pruritus and burning at the contact site are common symptoms.

Clinical course: if the offending agent is identified and removed, ACD and ICD subside. In chronic contact dermatitis, the presence or absence of sleep disturbance, the number and location of the involved sites, and the clinical course are indicators of disease severity. Superinfection may be a complication.

Diagnosis: if symptoms occur immediately after exposure, ICD should be considered. In ACD, patch tests can be useful to identify the agent to which the patient is allergic, while in ICD these are usually negative. Many patients may be sensitized to multiple allergens.

Therapy: it is important to establish the irritating/allergenic source so as to avoid further contact. Active dermatitis is usually treated with emollient creams, topical steroids, topical or oral antibiotics for secondary infection, oral steroids (usually short courses), azathioprine, ciclosporin or other immunosuppressive agents for severe cases. Tacrolimus ointment and pimecrolimus cream are immunomodulating drugs that inhibit calcineurin and may be helpful for ACD. Patients with active contact dermatitis in the genital area should avoid intercourse, as friction, spermicides, artificial lubricants, condoms, semen and vaginal secretions are all irritants.

Suggested Reading

Bhate K, Landeck L, Gonzalez E et al (2010) Genital contact dermatitis: a retrospective analysis. Dermatitis 21:317-20
Ljubojevi S, Lipozenci J, Celi D, Turci P (2009) Genital contact allergy. Acta Dermatovenerol Croat 17:285-8
Vermaat H, Smienk F, Rustemeyer T et al (2008) Anogenital allergic contact dermatitis, the role of spices and flavour allergy. Contact Dermatitis 59:233-7

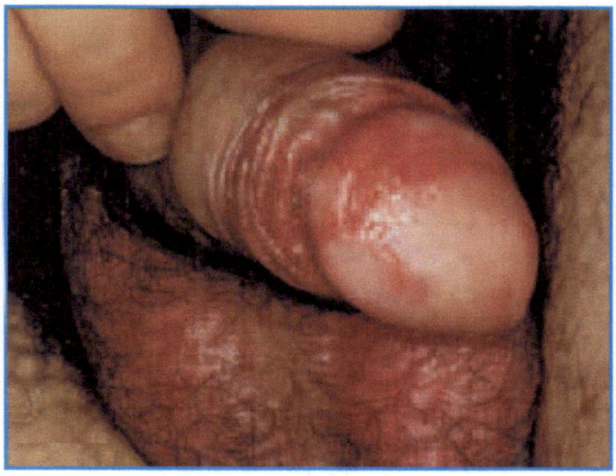

Fig. 5.1 Acute allergic contact dermatitis: intense erythema and oozing, involving the penis and the scrotum, caused by a topical cream

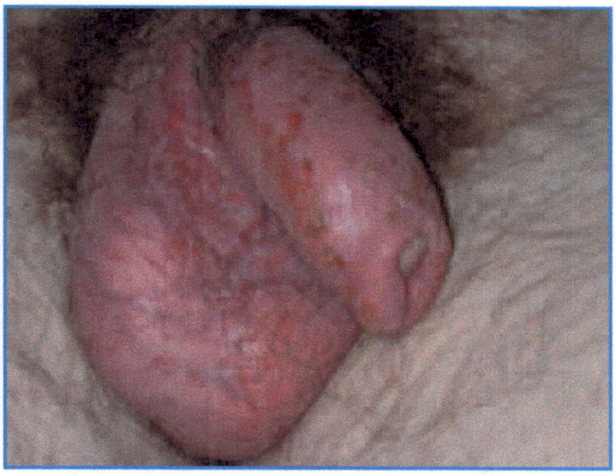

Fig. 5.2 Acute allergic contact dermatitis: erythema, vesicles, and crusts involving the penis and the scrotum after fragrance application

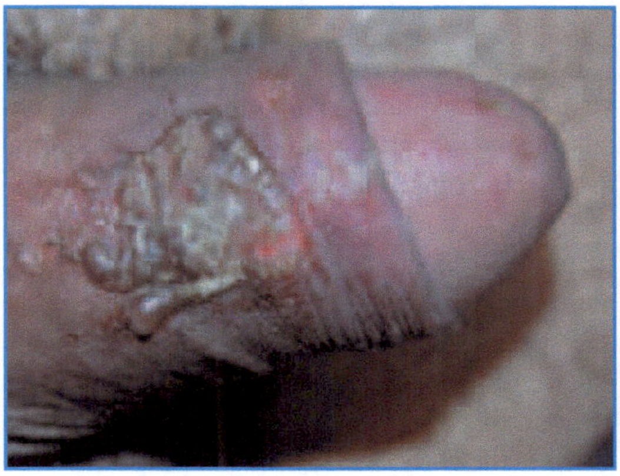

Fig. 5.3 Acute allergic contact dermatitis: blisters on the shaft due to topical medication

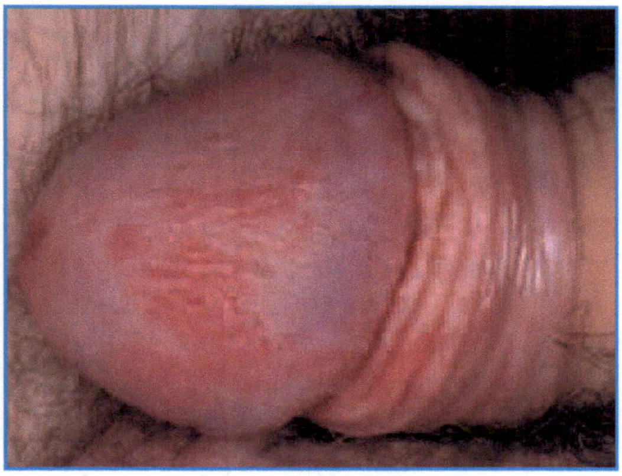

Fig. 5.4 Acute irritant contact dermatitis: slight erythema of the glans in an incontinent patient

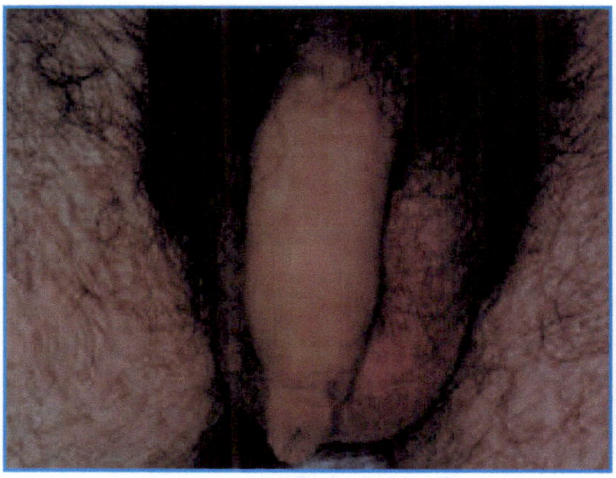

Fig. 5.5 Acute irritant contact dermatitis: slight erythema on the shaft due to condom use

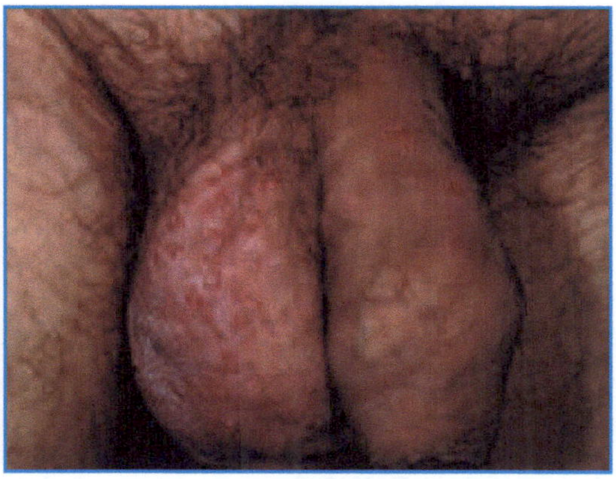

Fig. 5.6 Chronic irritant contact dermatitis: hyperkeratosis and lichenification of the penile and scrotal skin

Atopic Dermatitis

Definition: Atopic Dermatitis (AD) is a chronic, inflammatory, noninfective skin disease characterized by pruritus, eczema, xerosis (dry skin), and lichenification.

Etiology: it is a disease of unknown origin. A hereditary component of the disease has been recognized, as it is often seen in multiple members of the same family. Several factors may trigger or worsen atopic dermatitis, including dry skin, cold weather, exposure to aggressive detergents, tight clothing, and seasonal allergies.

Epidemiology: it is very common and its incidence and prevalence appear to be increasing. It is estimated that AD accounts for about 20% of all dermatologic referrals. Although quite difficult to establish, since the diagnostic criteria are not universally applied and standardized, its prevalence is thought to range from 10% to 30%. Localization on the penis and/or scrotum is rare.

Clinical appearance: although AD can occur at any age, it usually starts in early infancy. In the genital area the skin may become extremely itchy and inflamed. Repeated scratching may lead to crusting, scaling, lichenification, and hyperpigmentation.

Clinical course: it is a chronic disease that most often affects infants and young children. In some instances, it may persist into adulthood or first show up later in life. A large number of patients tend to have a long-term course with various episodes of exacerbation and remission.

Diagnosis: past medical history and clinical appearance generally prompt the correct diagnosis. Currently, there is no single specific diagnostic test.

Therapy: the primary treatment involves prevention, by avoiding or minimizing environmental triggers. Fingernails should be cut very short to avoid scratching. The use of soap should be discouraged because of its drying effect. Topical treatments (corticosteroid creams and ointments, antibiotics) can be used to reduce both the dryness and inflammation of the skin. Pimecrolimus cream and tacrolimus ointment are reasonable alternative options to corticosteroids. Oral antihistamines given in the early evening may be helpful in controlling nightime scratching.

Suggested Reading

Beltrani VS (2012) Atopic dermatitis in adults. Dermatitis 23:52-3
Cookson H, Smith C (2012) Systemic treatment of adult atopic dermatitis. Clin Med 12:172-6
Denby KS, Beck LA (2012) Update on systemic therapies for atopic dermatitis. Curr Opin Allergy Clin Immunol 12:421-6

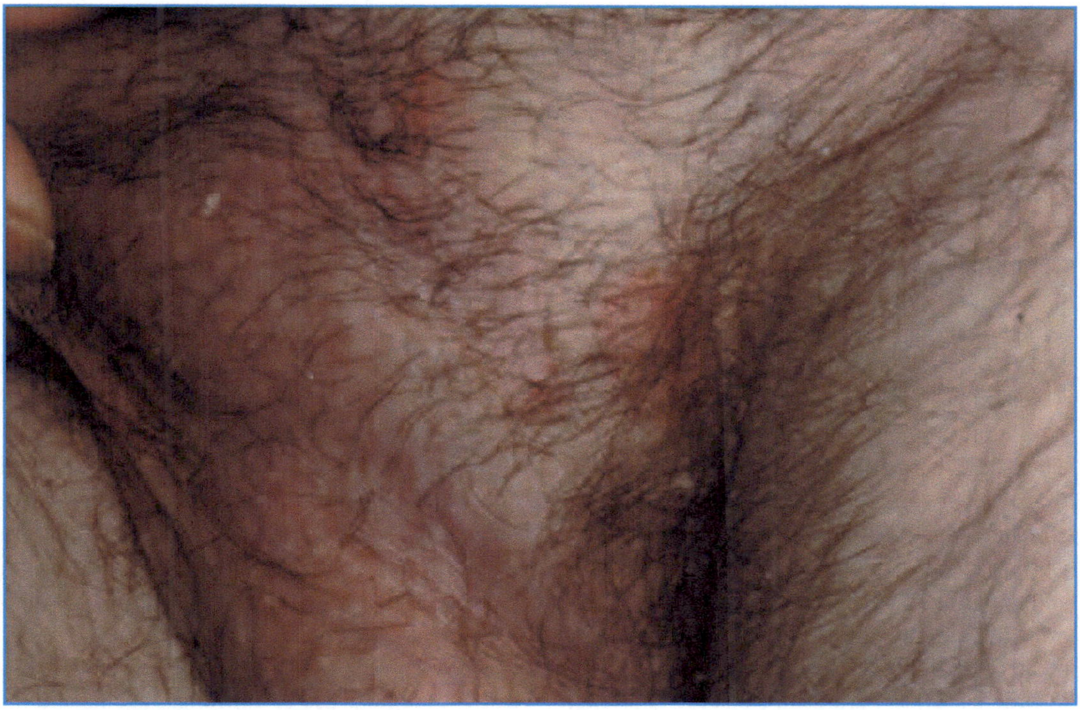

Fig. 5.7 Erythema and scaling of the scrotum

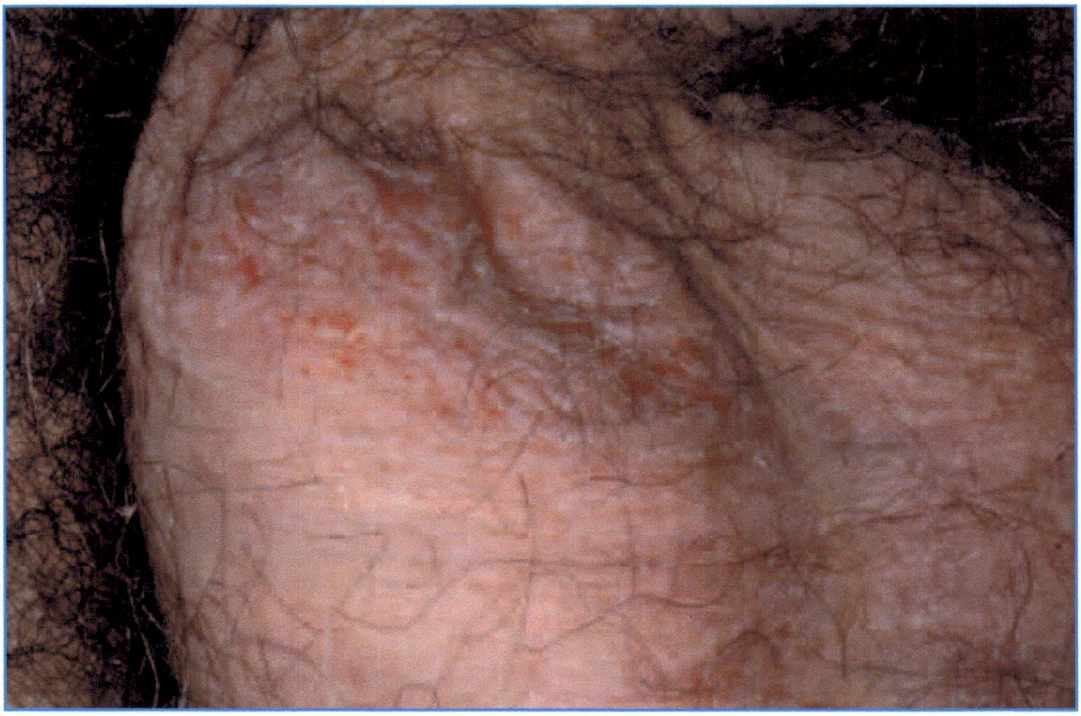

Fig. 5.8 Crusting, scaling, and lichenification of the scrotum

Seborrheic Dermatitis

Definition: Seborrheic Dermatitis (SD) is an inflammatory and nontransmissible disorder patterned on the sebum-rich areas of the body.

Etiology: its cause is unknown, but it is believed to be an inflammatory reaction related to a proliferation of a normal skin inhabitant, a yeast called *Malassezia furfur* (formerly known as *Pityrosporum ovale*). It may be worsened by seasonal climate changes in humidity and temperature as well as by illness, psychological stress, fatigue, and impairment of general health. It is more common in immunocompromised (especially HIV positive) or debilitated patients with neurological disorders such as Parkinson's disease or stroke.

Epidemiology: it is common, with a prevalence of about 1% to 2% in the general population. It is more frequent in men but its genital localization is more common in women.

Clinical appearance: erythematous marginated plaques with characteristic yellowish scaling are usually found. Genital lesions are usually observed in the context of a more generalized disease. If superinfection ensues, itching may worsen.

Clinical course: it is a chronic disorder, and there is usually no treatment that stops it permanently.

Diagnosis: it can be made based on the medical history and physical examination. Detection in other seborrheic areas is usually helpful to confirm diagnosis. When the diagnosis is unclear, a skin biopsy is suggested, although the histological findings are not specific.

Therapy: SD can generally be kept under control with regular use of antifungal agents and intermittent applications of low potency topical steroids. Creams, foams or lotions containing an antifungal agent, such as ketoconazole, reduce flare-ups, supporting the idea that the yeast is a contributing factor. In the hair-bearing genital skin a lotion is preferable.

Suggested Reading

Gaitanis G, Magiatis P, Hantschke M et al (2012) The Malassezia genus in skin and systemic diseases. Clin Microbiol Rev 25:106-41

Sampaio AL, Mameri AC, Vargas TJ et al (2011) Seborrheic dermatitis. An Bras Dermatol 86:1061-71

Schmidt JA (2011) Seborrheic dermatitis: a clinical practice snapshot. Nurse Pract 36:32-7

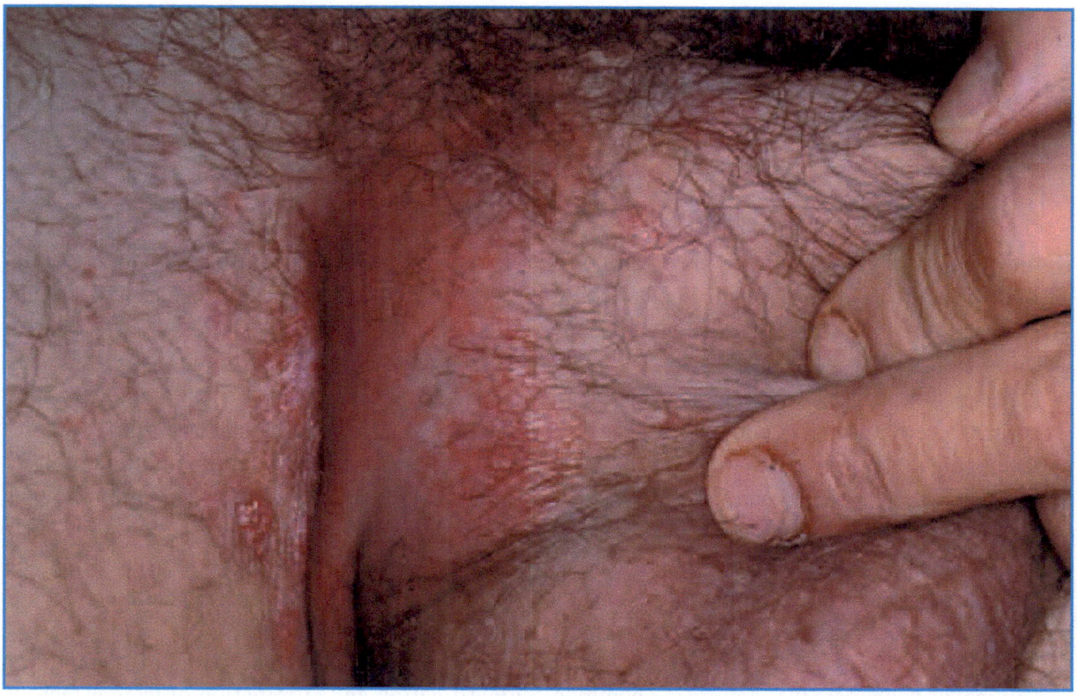

Fig. 5.9 Erythematous and oozing plaques involving the scrotum and the groin

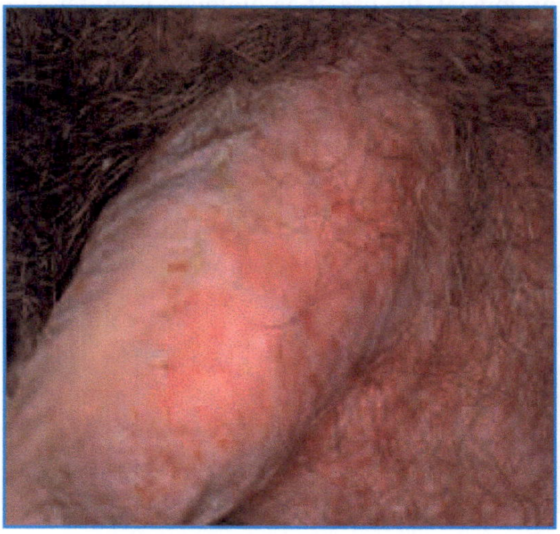

Fig. 5.10 Erythematous plaques of the penis with typical yellowish scales

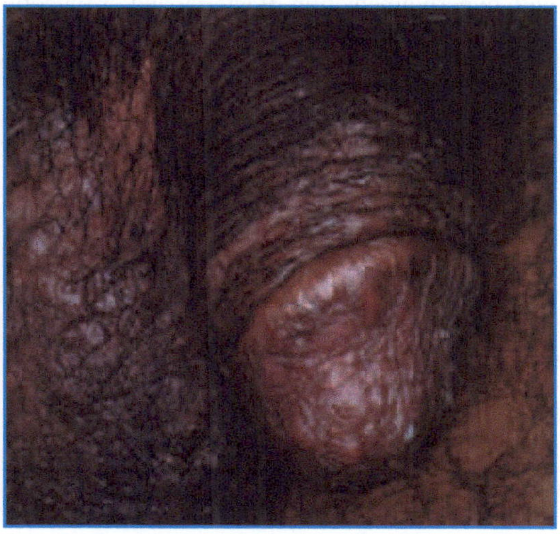

Fig. 5.11 Lichenification and hyperpigmentation of penis and scrotum in an Afro-American patient

Lichen Simplex (Neurodermatitis)

Definition: lichen simplex (neurodermatitis) is a chronic inflammatory disease in which itching gives rise to scratching and subsequent cutaneous inflammation.

Etiology: the exact cause remains unknown. Exposure to certain triggers can increase the risk of developing neurodermatitis. Stress and nervous tension increase itching. In young patients the disease is more often associated with anxiety, in the elderly with depression.

Epidemiology: it is a common disease that affects more women than men. It generally affects adults.

Clinical appearance: the scrotum is a common location. The disease starts insidiously and may result in one or many itchy patches. The affected area is erythematous with excoriations, often showing grouped small firm papules, or thickened skin with hyperpigmentation. Bacterial and/or mycotic superinfection may occur because of continuous scratching.

Clinical course: it tends to be very persistent, and it readily recurs despite initial treatment is often effective. Chronic itching and scratching can cause excoriations, lichenification and hyperpigmentations, and the disease results in a chronic "itch-scratch cycle".

Diagnosis: it may be difficult in earlier stages, since neurodermatitis may occur along with other common skin disorders, such as eczema and psoriasis. An anamnestic documentation of itch-scratch cycles and a clinical examination showing lichenification, with or without excoriations, help diagnosis. The diagnostic work up includes cultures for fungi and/or bacteria, patch testing, and a skin biopsy.

Therapy: successful treatment depends on identification and elimination of trigger factors, stopping the itch-scratch cycle. Over-the-counter and prescription creams can help ease neurodermatitis symptoms. A low-potency steroid cream would be appropriate, but if lichenification is prominent, the use of an ointment is preferable. Moisturizing creams are also recommended. Oral antihistamines are indicated in the early evening to control nighttime scratching. In elderly patients the use of antidepressants should be considered.

Suggested Reading

Kapp A, Werfel T (2006) Neurodermatitis. Hautarzt 57:566

Lichon V, Khachemoune A (2007) Lichen simplex chronicus. Dermatol Nurs 19:276

Prajapati V, Barankin B (2008) Dermacase. Lichen simplex chronicus. Can Fam Physician 54:1391-3

Rajalakshmi R, Thappa DM, Jaisankar TJ, Nath AK (2011) Lichen simplex chronicus of anogenital region: a clinico-etiological study. Indian J Dermatol Venereol Leprol 77:28-36

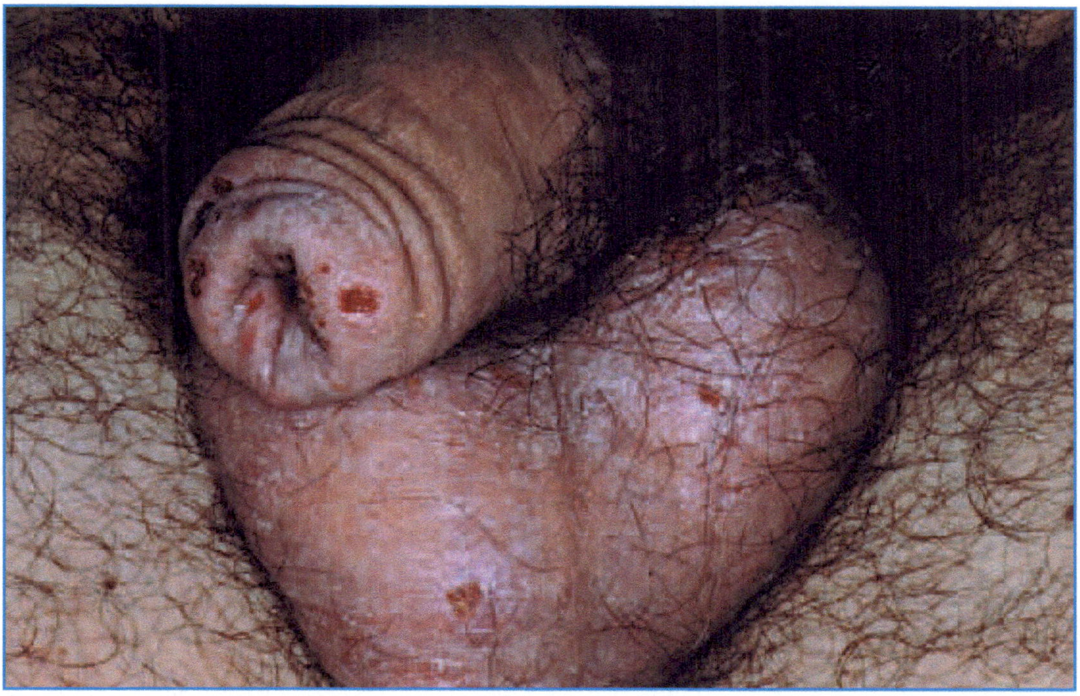

Fig. 5.12 Lichenification and excoriations involving the penis and the scrotum

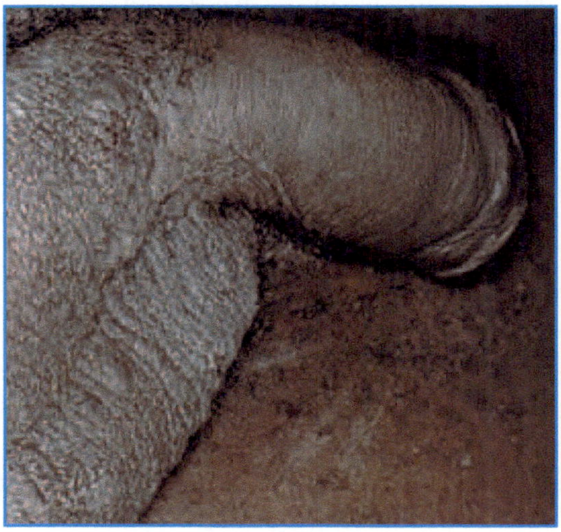

Fig. 5.13 Lichenification of the scrotum in an Afro-American patient

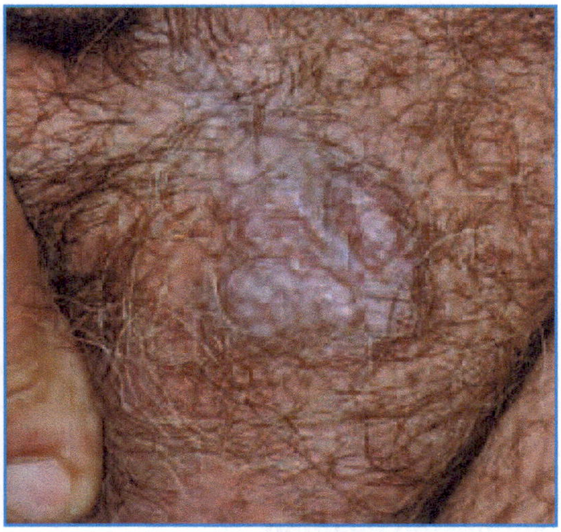

Fig. 5.14 Lichenification of scrotal skin

Psoriasis

Definition: psoriasis is a chronic, inflammatory, noncontagious erythemato-squamous disease.

Etiology: it is unknown. In predisposed patients, trigger factors such as stress and local trauma can favor the appearance or worsening of skin lesions. Koebner's phenomenon may play a role in the location of the psoriasis in the genital area because of local irritation produced by continuous friction from clothing, harsh hygiene products, and/or sexual intercourse.

Epidemiology: the prevalence in the general population is approximately 3%. The genital skin is involved in 29–40% of patients. In many cases, genital psoriasis is part of a more generalized plaque psoriasis or occurs in the setting of inverse psoriasis. Psoriasis is located exclusively in the genital area in only 2–5% of psoriatic patients.

Clinical appearance: both scrotum and shaft may be affected, but the glans is the most commonly affected area. Occasionally, the whole penis, scrotum, and inguinal folds are involved. Psoriatic lesions on the genital area are brightly erythematous, often less well-demarcated and devoid of the typical psoriatic scales, due to maceration. Whereas in uncircumcised males the nonscaling plaques are most common under the prepuce and on the proximal glans, in circumcised male patients they are usually present on the glans and corona, and they may be more scaly than those usually seen in genital skin. Fissures, pruritus, and/or burning in the affected area, ranging from minimal to marked, may be observed.

Clinical course: genital psoriasis is a chronic disease that exhibits ups and downs. It is usually controlled by the prevention of local traumas and the use of adequate treatments. Patients with genital psoriasis often experience emotional stress and have difficulty coping with the disease.

Diagnosis: it can usually be made clinically. The genitals may be the only affected area, but lesions are more often part of a more generalized disorder. In the case of aspecific genital lesions, the diagnosis may be suggested by the presence of typical lesions elsewhere, or nail deformities, or joint complaints. Videodermatoscopy may be helpful in addressing the correct diagnosis: at low magnifications (X10–X50) a dotted pattern is evident; higher magnifications (X100-X400) are able to visualize dilated, elongated and convoluted capillaries showing a typical "*glomerular*" or "*bushy*" pattern. Skin biopsy is needed in the case of single and/or difficult to diagnose lesions.

Therapy: in patients with exclusively genital lesions, topical therapy can be sufficient. It is better to avoid irritant topicals in the management of genital psoriasis, as they can worsen symptoms. First-line therapy includes low- and mid-potency topical corticosteroids, which may be used in combination with topical vitamin D analogues (calcipotriol). Pimecrolimus ointment or tacrolimus

Suggested Reading

Lacarrubba F, Nasca MR, Micali G (2009) Videodermatoscopy enhances diagnostic capability in psoriatic balanitis. J Am Acad Dermatol 61:1084-6

Meeuwis KA, De Hullu JA, De Jager ME et al (2010) Genital psoriasis: a questionnaire-based survey on a concealed skin disease in the Netherlands. J Eur Acad Dermatol Venereol 24:1425-30

Meeuwis KA, de Hullu JA, Massuger LF et al (2011) Genital psoriasis: A systematic literature review on this hidden skin disease. Acta Derm Venereol 91:5-11

Meeuwis KA, De Hullu JA, Van De Nieuwenhof HP et al (2011) Quality of life and sexual health in patients with genital psoriasis. Br J Dermatol 164:1247-55

cream may be useful, though they may cause local irritation and stinging. UVB and PUVA therapy is not recommended to treat genital psoriatic lesions because of the high risk of penile or scrotal squamous cell carcinoma. Systemic treatment is indicated in case of generalized psoriasis. Local hygiene is very important as local maceration and continuous use of corticosteroids can enhance the risk of bacterial and/or fungal superinfections, especially in the intertriginous areas.

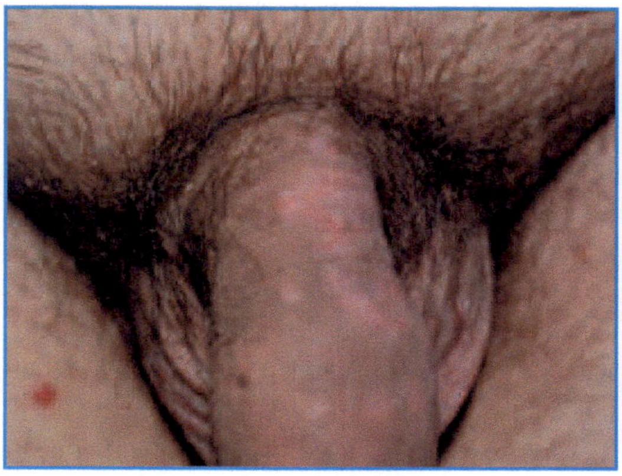

Fig. 5.15 Typical erythematous and scaling plaques on the penis

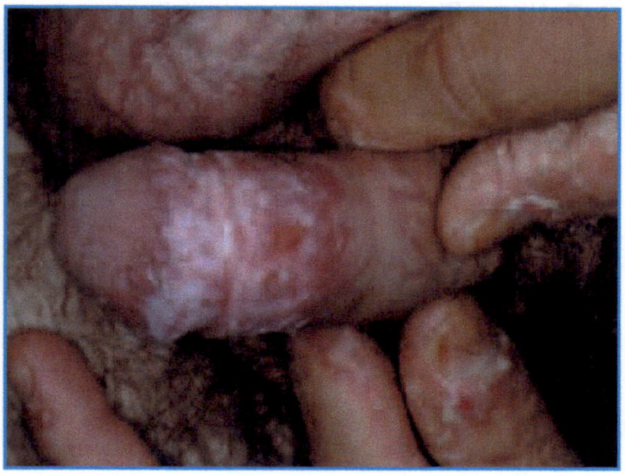

Fig. 5.16 Typical erythematous and scaling plaques involving the penis and the fingers in an HIV+ patient

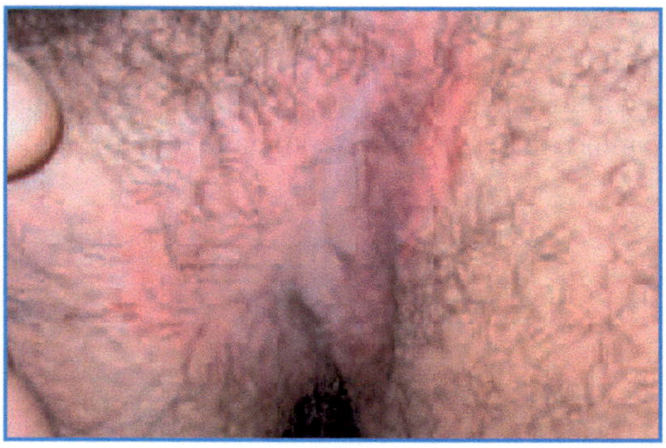

Fig. 5.17 Inverse psoriasis: typical erythematous and oozing plaque of the groin

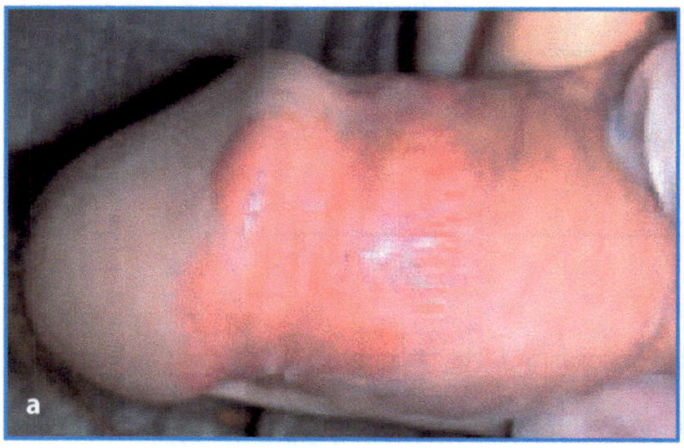

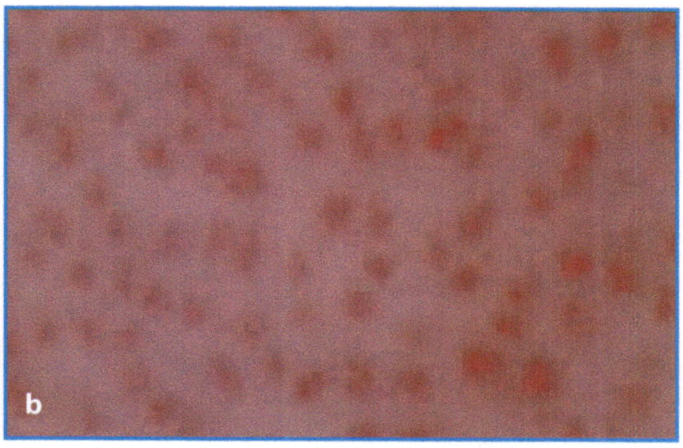

Fig. 5.18 Psoriatic balanitis. **a** Erythematous and scaling plaques of the penis. **b** Videodermatoscopy (X200) showing dilated, elongated, and convoluted capillaries with a typical "bushy" pattern

Pityriasis Rosea (Gibert)

Definition: Pityriasis Rosea (PR) is a common inflammatory disease with characteristic skin findings.

Etiology: it is unknown. Infectious agents (*Mycoplasma hominis, Staphylococcus albus, spirochaetes, beta-hemolytic Streptococcus*), drugs, and environmental factors have been implicated in its pathogenesis. Current evidence indicates that PR exanthema may possibly be linked to a human herpes virus infection.

Epidemiology: its incidence ranges between 0.4% and 4.8%. It is most common in young adults, and usually occurs in spring and autumn.

Clinical appearance: it is characterized by erythematosquamous lesions usually confined to the trunk and to the upper third of the arms and legs. The lesions on the genital area represent part of the general eruption. The rash starts with a "herald patch" that precedes the onset of other similar smaller lesions. The herald patch is a solitary large lesion which occurs in half of the patients. When it occurs in the genital area, it may resemble tinea. The smaller lesions that ensue are roundish, salmon-colored, slightly scaling, especially at their edge, and show a typical pattern on the trunk ("Christmas tree rash"). The rash is generally asymptomatic, but occasionally may be intensely itchy.

Clinical course: it is benign and the lesions usually disappear spontaneously after 6 to 8 weeks, without scarring or residual pigmentation. A recurrence may be observed in about 5% of patients.

Diagnosis: it is based on the clinical appearance and examination of other skin areas, such as trunk and arms. In some atypical cases a syphilis serologic test, culture, or skin biopsy may be required to rule out other disorders.

Therapy: it usually resolves spontaneously and treatment is not required. The use of mild soaps is recommended. In presence of itching, oral antihistamines may provide symptomatic relief.

Suggested Reading

Rebora A, Drago F, Broccolo F (2010) Pityriasis rosea and herpesviruses: facts and controversies. Clin Dermatol 28: 497-501

Sonthalia S, Singal A, Pandhi D, Singh UR (2011) Annular purpuric eruption in an adult male. Indian J Dermatol Venereol Leprol 77:731

Wyndham M (2008) Pityriasis rosea. Community Pract 81:16

Zawar V (2010) Giant Pityriasis Rosea. Indian J Dermatol 55:192–4

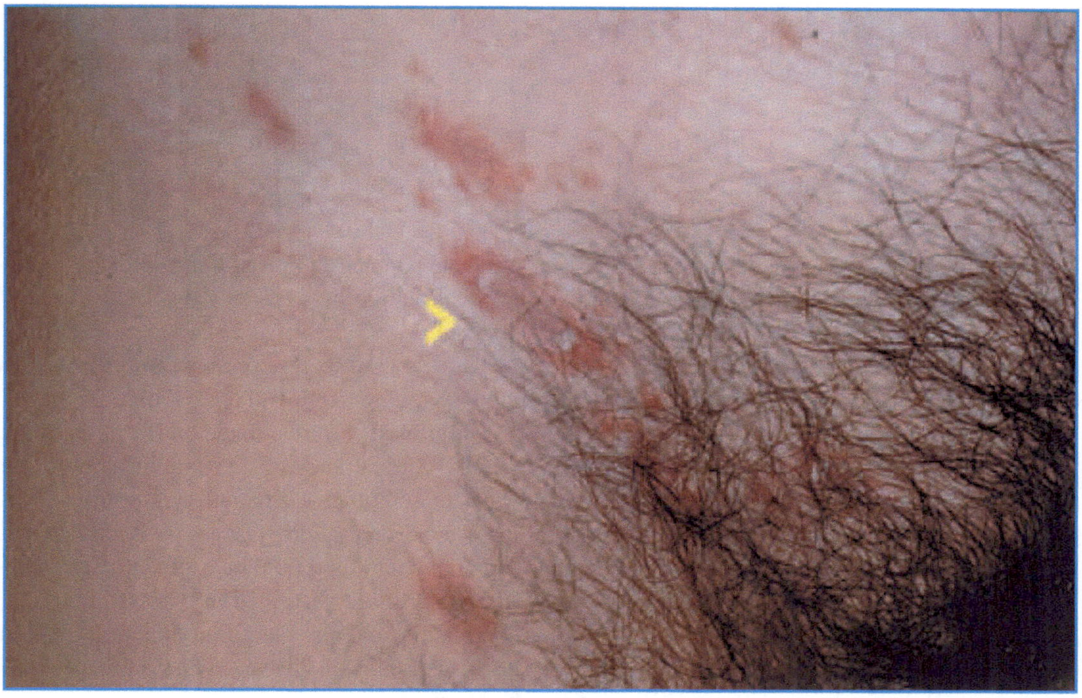

Fig. 5.19 “Herald patch” in the genital area

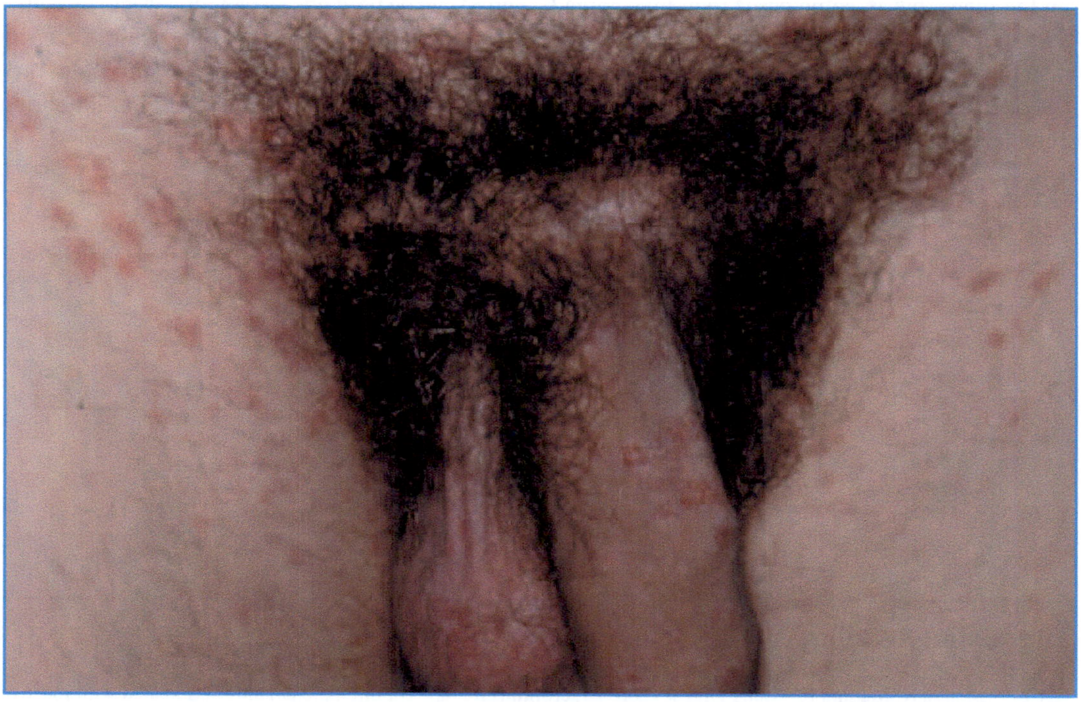

Fig. 5.20 Typical roundish, erythematous, and scaling lesions involving the penis and the groin

Circinate Reactive Balanitis (Reiter's Disease)

Definition: circinate reactive balanitis is a marker for, or associated with, Reiter's syndrome, a disorder characterized by the triad of symptoms (conjunctivitis, urethritis, and arthritis) occurring after an infection, mostly of the urogenital or gastrointestinal tract.

Etiology: there is an association with the HLA B27 gene in 60-80% of cases. *Chlamydia trachomatis* is implicated in 70% of cases. Other associated infections include those caused by enteric pathogens, such as *Salmonella*, *Shigella*, *Yersinia* and *Campylobacter*.

Epidemiology: it occurs in 20-80% of male patients with Reiter's disease. Reiter's disease is more frequent in men, although cases have also been reported in children and women.

Clinical appearance: the lesions usually occur on the glans, but in some cases they may spread over the corona and foreskin. In circumcised patients they appear as erythematous, well-demarcated, scaling or crusted plaques, while in uncircumcised patients they appear as small white circinate papules and resembling single or multiple coalescing rings. Palms and soles are usually affected.

Clinical course: it is a chronic disorder that requires ongoing treatment.

Diagnosis: it can be made on the basis of the clinical appearance. The patient should be checked for other signs and symptoms of Reiter's syndrome and/or psoriasis. Bacterial and candidal balanitis should be excluded. Stool cultures should be performed in those with enteric complaints, and any identified infections should be treated. In inconclusive cases, skin biopsy may be required.

Therapy: low-potency corticosteroid creams applied 1-2 times daily usually produce a prompt response. If not, a mid- to high-potency corticosteroid can be used once a day for a week. Systemic involvement (reactive arthritis, uveitis) can be managed with nonsteroidal anti-inflammatory drugs, sulfasalazine, methotrexate, azathioprine or anti-TNF-alpha medications.

Suggested Reading

Herrera-Esparza R, Medina F, Avalos-Díaz E (2009) Tacrolimus therapy for circinate balanitis associated with reactive arthritis. J Clin Rheumatol 15:377-9

Serrano-Grau P, Ferrando J (2007) Reiter's syndrome. Med Clin (Barc) 128:400

Wu IB, Schwartz RA (2008) Reiter's syndrome: the classic triad and more. J Am Acad Dermatol 59:113-21

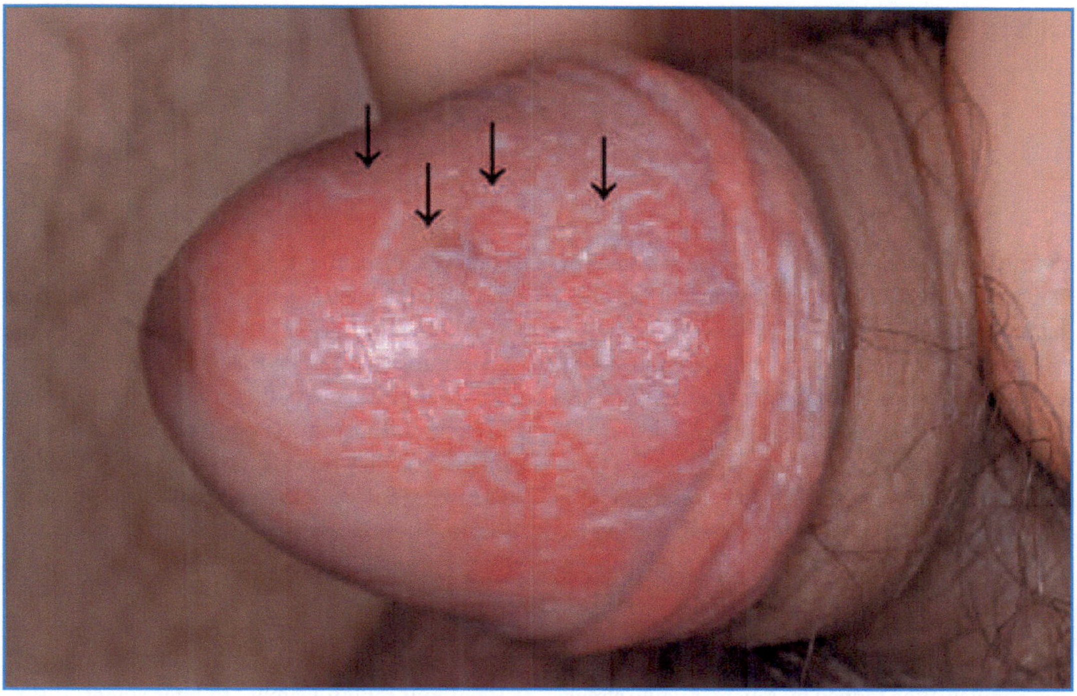

Fig. 5.21 Typical erythematous and circinate (*arrows*) plaques on the glans

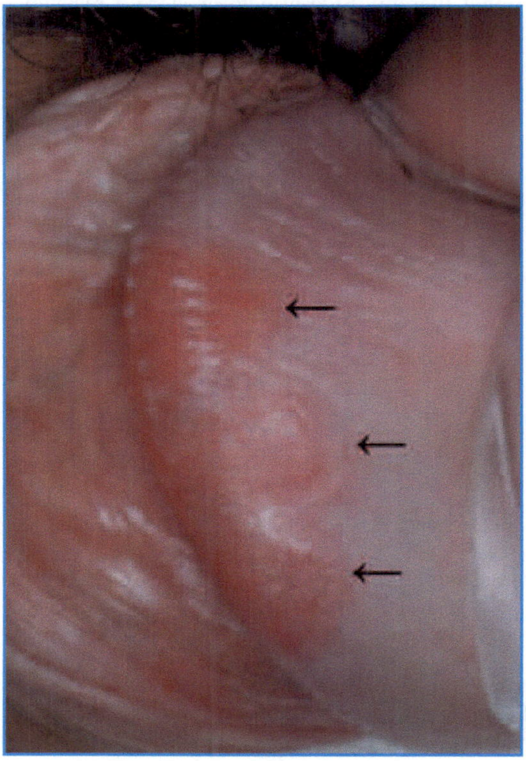

Fig. 5.22 Typical erythematous, sharply marginated, and circinate plaques involving the glans and the coronal sulcus

Lichen Planus

Definition: Lichen Planus (LP) is a chronic, inflammatory, mucocutaneous disease that can affect the mucosae.

Etiology: it is unknown, although many studies have investigated and supported an autoimmune pathogenesis. Lymphocytes, particularly T-cells, play a major role.

Epidemiology: genital lesions are frequent in patients with LP. It has been estimated that approximately 25% of men with cutaneous LP have genital lesions, but isolated genital LP is unusual.

Clinical appearance: the lesions usually appear on the glans as well-defined lilac annular pruritic papules often topped by reticular white streaks known as Wickham's striae. In many, but not all, Wickham's striae may also be detected in the oral mucosa. Genital lichen planus may also exhibit other morphologic variants (hypertrophic and erosive). Erosive forms may be very painful, and, in longstanding cases, may lead to penile disfigurement. Erosive LP is usually not associated with cutaneous lesions, but oral involvement can be present.

Clinical course: non-erosive forms are well controlled with therapy. Erosive LP is poorly responsive to treatment, it is chronic and painful, causing considerable discomfort and impaired sexual function.

Diagnosis: it can be made on the basis of the clinical appearance. In the case of unspecific features, careful inspection of other skin areas or of oral mucosa may provide the diagnostic clue. Dermatoscopy ensures easy and rapid recognition of Wickham's striae, which appear as pearly whitish structures which secondarily develop thin spikes (*comblike projections*) or arboriform ramifications departing from the periphery. Skin biopsy is indicated in inconclusive cases of subtle erosive LP without mouth lesions. In later stages, differential diagnosis between LP and lichen sclerosus may be very difficult. Moreover, both diseases may sometimes coexist in a single patient.

Therapy: a potent topical steroid is the conventional therapy. Side-effects or steroid resistance can be encountered, and a second-line therapy such as topical pimecrolimus may be required. In severe forms, systemic therapy with oral prednisone or cyclosporine can be used. Patient education and support is encouraged.

Suggested Reading

Badri T, Kenani N, Benmously R et al (2011) Isolated genital annular lichen planus. Acta Dermatovenerol Alp Panonica Adriat 20:31-3

Hidalgo ER, Nicolás GM, Muñoz AA et al (2007) Unknown origin fever and lichen planus in penis. An Med Interna 24:356-7

Lonsdale-Eccles AA, Velangi S (2005) Topical pimecrolimus in the treatment of genital lichen planus: a prospective case series. Br J Dermatol 153:390-4

Usatine RP, Tinitigan M (2011) Diagnosis and treatment of lichen planus. Am Pham Physician 84:53-60

Vázquez-López F (2010) Lichen ruber planus. In: Micali G, Lacarrubba F (eds). Dermatoscopy in clinical practice: beyond pigmented lesions. Informa Healthcare Ltd, London (UK)

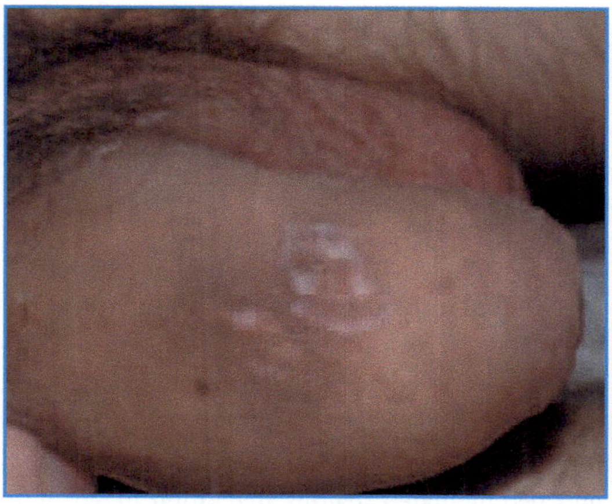

Fig. 5.23 Typical lilac papules, covered by reticular, white streaks (Wickham's striae), on the shaft

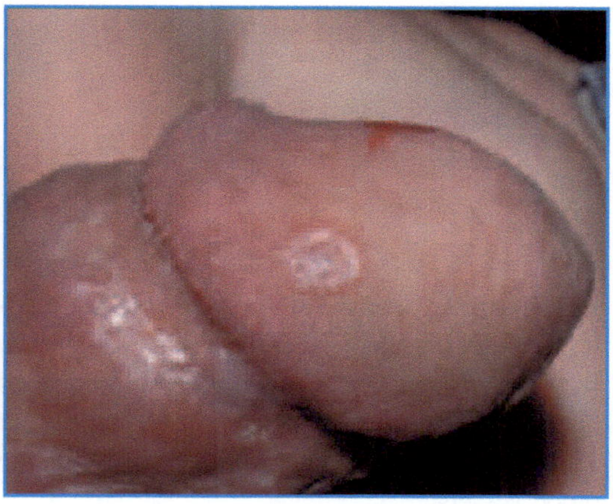

Fig. 5.24 Single annular papule on the glans

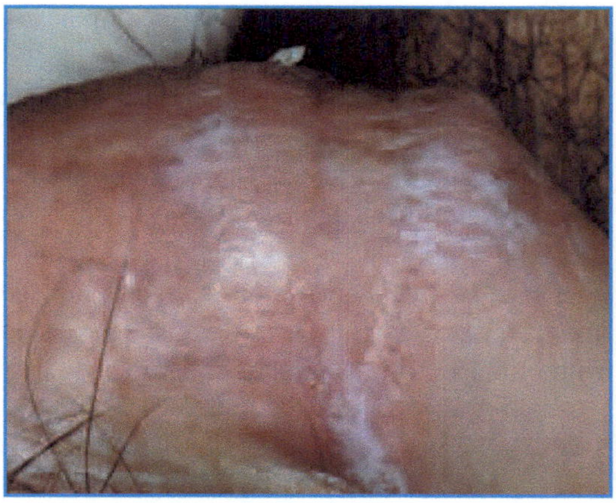

Fig. 5.25 Coalescent papules, with evident Wickham's striae, involving the glans and the foreskin

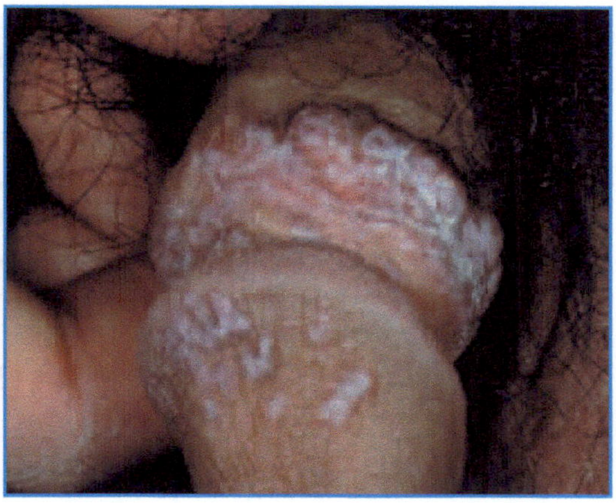

Fig. 5.26 Hypertrophic lichen planus: whitish and verrucous papules on the glans and foreskin

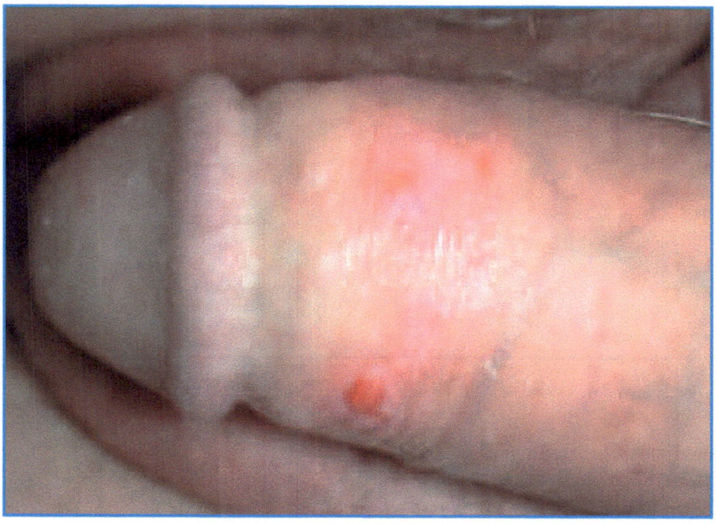

Fig. 5.27 Erosive lichen planus: ulcerative lesions on the foreskin

Pyogenic Granuloma

Definition: Pyogenic Granuloma (PG) is a common benign vascular lesion of the skin and mucosa. It is not an infective, purulent or granulomatous disease, as the name might suggest, but it is rather a reactive inflammatory process involving the blood vessels.

Etiology: it is not fully understood. Rapid growth occurs in response to an unknown stimulus that triggers endothelial proliferation and angiogenesis. Trauma and burns can sometimes be the causative agents, but frequently there is no identifiable cause. Other suggested precipitating factors include infection, hormonal influences (pregnancy and oral contraceptive pill in women), and cytogenetic abnormalities. PG has also been associated with the intake of some medications, such as systemic and topical retinoids, protease inhibitors, and chemotherapeutic agents.

Epidemiology: its incidence decreases with age, and it peaks at 6-7 years.

Clinical appearance: on the scrotum and penis it appears as a solitary, red, purple or yellowish papule or nodule arising from normal skin. Size varies from a few millimeters to several centimeters in diameter. PGs are friable, polypoid and pedunculated lesions that often bleed, with consequent pain, crusting or ulceration.

Clinical course: rapid eruption and growth occur over a few weeks. Untreated lesions spontaneously involute, but only a minority completely clear with residual atrophy within six months. Recurrence rates following treatment can be quite high (40-50%).

Diagnosis: it is usually made on clinical grounds, and histopathology is only seldom required in doubtful cases.

Therapy: treatment options include curettage and cautery, cryotherapy, shave excision, excision with primary closure, and laser therapy.

Suggested Reading

Abdul Gaffoor PM (1998) Pyogenic granuloma of the scrotum. Cutis 62:282

Eickhorst KM, Nurzia MJ, Barone JG (2003) Pediatric pyogenic granuloma of the glans penis. Urology 61:644

Tomasini C, Puiatti P, Bernengo MG (1998) Multiple pyogenic granuloma of the penis. Sex Transm Infect 74:221-2

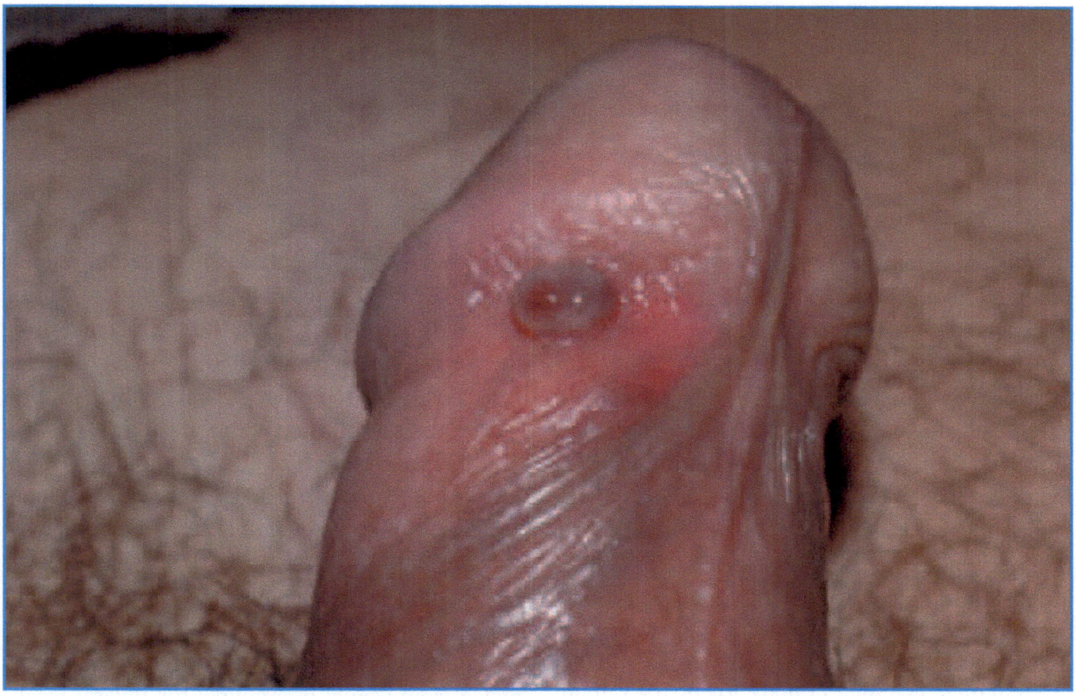

Fig. 5.28 Circumscribed, raised, and reddish nodule arising from the coronal sulcus

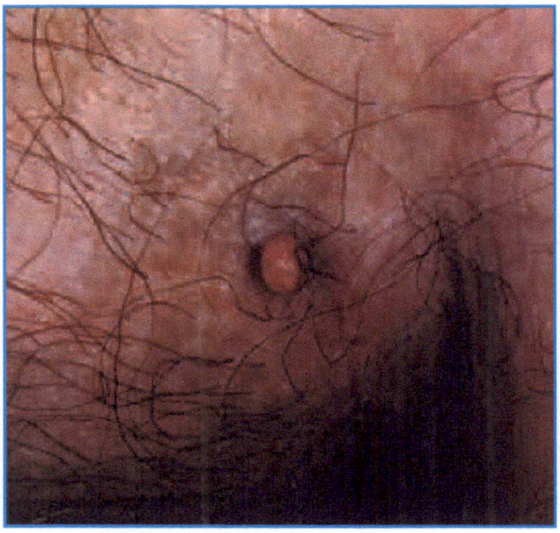

Fig. 5.29 Small, raised, and reddish nodule on the scrotum

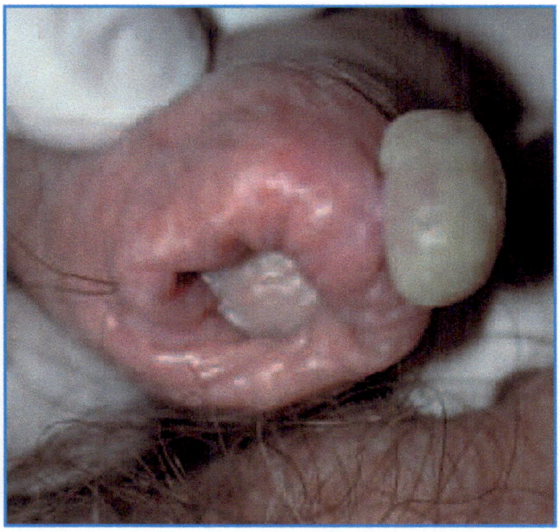

Fig. 5.30 Pedunculated and whitish nodule arising from the foreskin

Sclerosing Lymphangitis

Definition: Sclerosing Lymphangitis (SL) is an inflammation of the lymphatic channels proximal to the glans, producing a cord-like thickening.

Etiology: it is unknown. Circumferential scarring from circumcision, enterovirus infection, tuberculosis are some of the postulated etiologies. However, the most frequent hypothetic triggering factor is a local mechanical trauma from repeated penile injury during vigorous sexual intercourse. In 25% of all reported cases, a close temporal relationship to gonorrhea, chlamydia, and syphilis has been noted.

Epidemiology: SL of the penis is usually seen in sexually active men in their 20s to 40s following sexual intercourse or masturbation.

Clinical appearance: it is characterized by a serpiginous, translucent, flesh-colored or reddish cord-like thickening, non-adherent to overlying skin and located on the shaft or glans, encircling the coronal sulcus parallel to the corona. Although it is mostly asymptomatic, some patients report pain and discomfort on erection.

Clinical course: it causes negligible physical discomfort to the patient and seems to resolve spontaneously within a relatively short period (4-6 weeks).

Diagnosis: it is usually made based on the clinical findings.

Therapy: the condition is self-limiting. Abstinence from sexual intercourse for several weeks with reassurance is the treatment of choice. Excision is rarely required in case of persistence.

Suggested Reading

Kumar B, Narang T, Radotra BD, Gupta S (2005) Mondor's disease of penis: a forgotten disease. Sex Transm Infect 81:480-2

Rosen T, Hwong H (2003) Sclerosing lymphangitis of the penis. J Am Acad Dermatol 49:916-8

Yap FB (2009) Nonvenereal sclerosing lymphangitis of the penis. South Med J 102:1269-71

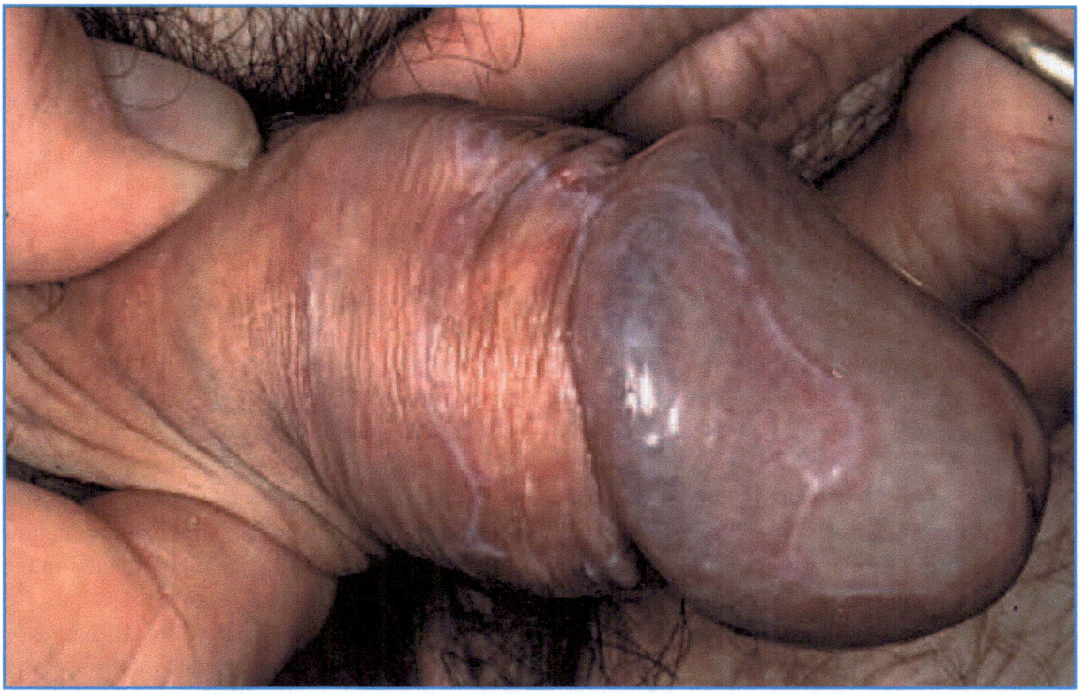

Fig. 5.31 Serpiginous, translucent, and reddish cord-like thickening on the glans and foreskin

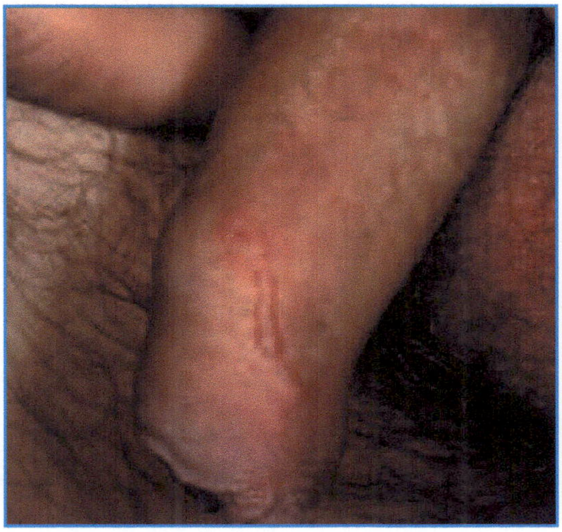

Fig. 5.32 Serpiginous and skin-colored tract on the shaft

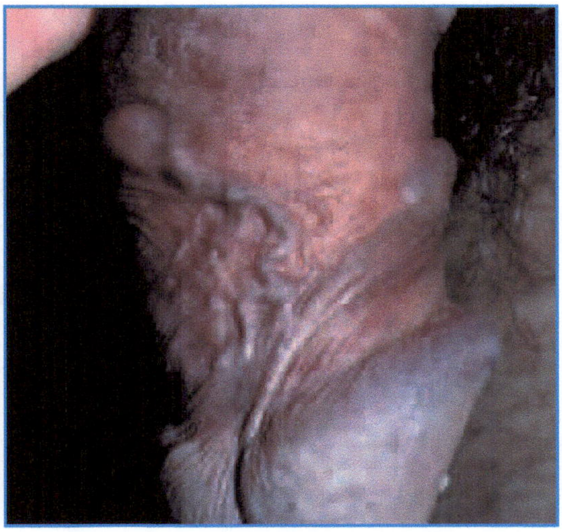

Fig. 5.33 Serpiginous and bluish tract on the ventral appearance of the shaft

Hidradenitis Suppurativa (Verneuil's Disease)

Definition: Hidradenitis Suppurativa (HS), also known as Verneuil's disease or acne inversa, is a chronic, inflammatory, suppurating, fistulizing, and scar-producing disorder affecting body areas that contain sweat glands.

Etiology: its exact cause is disputed. Traditionally considered to be a disease of the apocrine glands, it has been hypothesised to derive from a defect of the follicular epithelium. Some studies have suggested an autosomal dominant inheritance. Triggering factors possibly associated with HS include heat, humidity, and friction from clothing, obesity via occlusion and maceration, hyperandrogenism, chemical irritants, smoking, and lithium exposure. Bacterial infection is thought to occur secondarily.

Epidemiology: its precise incidence is uncertain. The disorder might be more common than once thought, since its diagnosis is frequently ignored or missed.

Clinical appearance: it mostly occurs in the armpits, groin, and buttocks, but the scalp may also be involved (dissecting folliculitis). Less severe cases may only present as a cluster of 2 or 3 deeply interconnected blackheads. Once the disease begins, it gets progressively worse. Extensive, deep inflammation leads to painful abscesses and fistulae that heal incompletely and cause cord-like scars on the skin. This condition can cause considerable discomfort to patients, hamper movements of the affected area and significantly impair the quality of life.

Clinical course: it is a chronic disabling disorder progressing relentlessly and leading to draining sinuses, fistulas, abscesses and progressive scarring. Other potential complications include dermal contraction, local or disseminated infection, and lymphedema.

Diagnosis: it is primarily clinical, based on the presence of both sinus tracts and abscesses with a characteristic distribution.

Therapy: it is difficult. In the early and mild stages, before extensive scarring develops, conservative measures such as warm baths, hydrotherapy, cryotherapy and topical cleansing agents to reduce the bacterial load may be useful. In moderate to severe cases, other treatment options, such as systemic antibiotics (erythromycin, tetracycline, minocycline, doxycycline), isotretinoin or steroid injection (normally combined with other treatments) are necessary. Local surgical excision should be performed as early as possible if abscesses, fistulas, scars, or sinus tracts occur.

Suggested Reading

Alikhan A, Lynch PJ, Eisen DB (2009) Hidradenitis suppurativa: a comprehensive review. J Am Acad Dermatol 60:539

Jemec GBE, Heidenheim M, Nielsen NH (1996) The prevalence of hidradenitis suppurativa and its potential precursor lesions. J Am Acad Dermatol 35:191-4

Jansen T, Altmeyer P, Plewig G (2001) Acne inversa (alias hidradenitis suppurativa). J Eur Acad Dermatol Venereol 15:532-40

Jansen T, Plewig G (2000) What's new in acne inversa (alias hidradenitis suppurativa)? J Eur Acad Dermatol Venereol 14(5):342-3

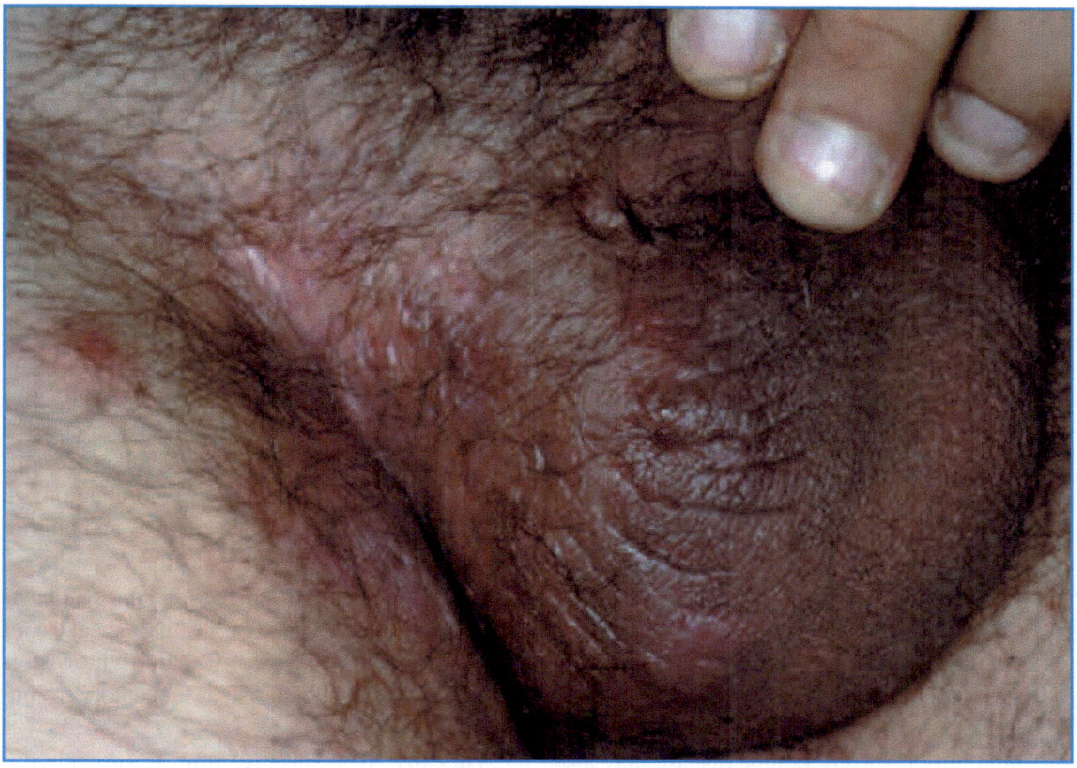

Fig. 5.34 Intense inflammation of the groin and scrotum with presence of deep nodules and scars

Erythema Multiforme

Definition: Erythema Multiforme (EM) is an acute, inflammatory skin disorder resulting from an immune response to antigenic sensitization.

Etiology: it is unknown but the disease is considered to be a type IV hypersensitivity reaction, usually associated with viral infections (herpes simplex virus), and medications (carbamazepine, phenytoin, sulfonamide, and penicillin). Other trigger factors include lymphoreticular malignancies and autoimmune diseases (lupus erythematosus and rheumatoid arthritis).

Epidemiology: globally, its frequency is estimated at approximately 1.2 - 6 cases per million individuals per year.

Clinical appearance: the penis and scrotum are commonly involved, but the disease may also occur elsewhere. Initially, erosions are located at the meatus and then extend to the glans and prepuce. Sometimes, the entire genitalia can be affected. In some cases, the disease occurs in the genital and oral mucosa without generalized cutaneous involvement. These patients are acutely ill. EM is often accompanied by fever, malaise and myalgias.

Clinical course: after bullous eruptions and erosions, the patient's condition gradually improves. Recurrences are possible after repeated drug exposure or following recurrent herpes simplex virus infection. Common complications in male genital areas are meatal stenosis and phimosis. Severe EM may result in death.

Diagnosis: it is based mainly on anamnesis and clinical appearance. Careful inspection of other skin areas as well as of the oral mucosa is recommended. A skin biopsy is mandatory to confirm the diagnosis.

Therapy: if a causative drug is suspected, it must be withdrawn as soon as possible. The use of systemic corticosteroids is debatable, but topical corticosteroids may be considered in treating genital EM. Local genital care is very important to prevent complications.

Suggested Reading

Borchers AT, Lee JL, Naguwa SM et al (2008) Stevens-Johnson syndrome and toxic epidermal necrolysis. Autoimmun Rev 7:598-605

Hazin R, Ibrahimi OA, Hazin MI, Kimyai-Asadi A (2008) Stevens-Johnson syndrome: pathogenesis, diagnosis, and management. Ann Med 40:129-38

Katoulis AC, Liakou A, Bozi E et al (2010) Erythema multiforme following vaccination for human papillomavirus. Dermatology 220:60-2

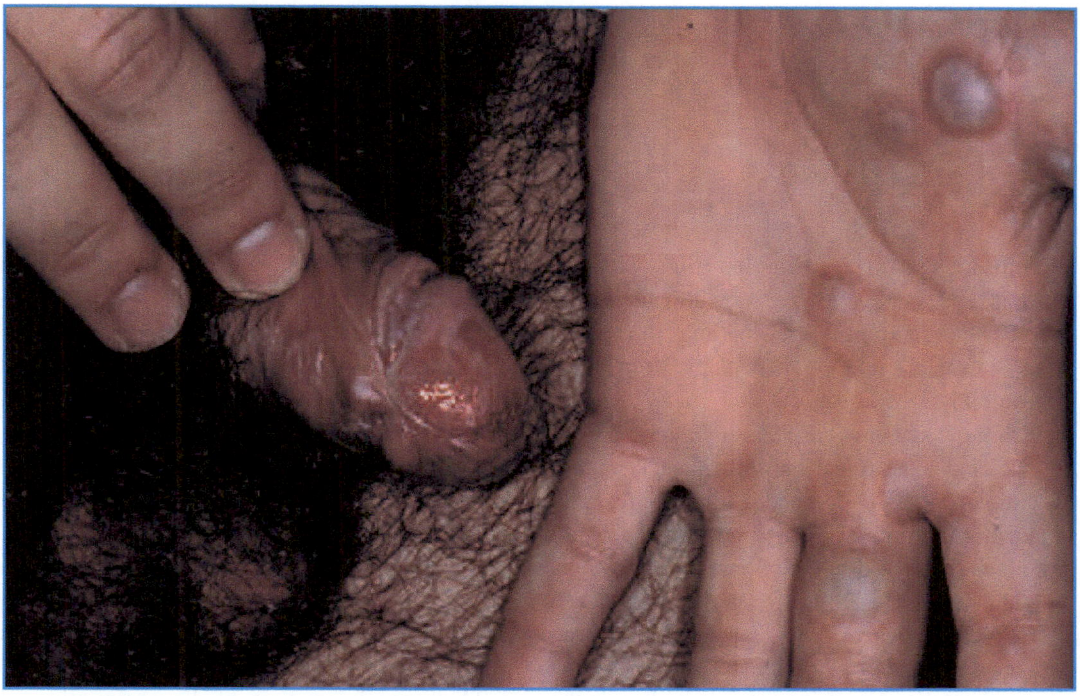

Fig. 5.35 Diffuse erosion of the glans with typical target-like bullous lesions on the palms

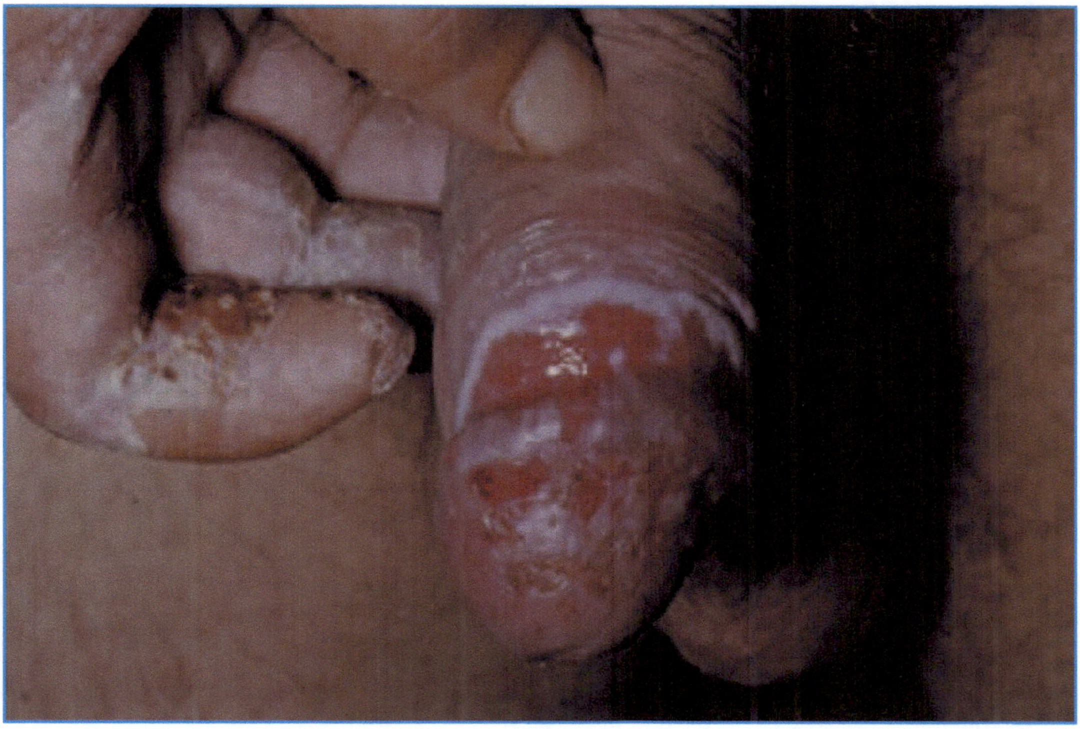

Fig. 5.36 Erosions and crusts involving the glans and foreskin

Fixed Drug Eruption

Definition: Fixed Drug Eruption (FDE) is a mucocutaneous reaction to a systemic drug characterized by the recurrent onset of skin lesions at the same sites each time the responsible drug is administered.

Etiology: any drug can cause FDE, notably antibiotics and nonsteroidal anti-inflammatory agents, by a direct cytotoxic immune-mediated effect.

Epidemiology: it is quite frequent, representing about 10% of drug reactions. The penis is a frequent site for FDE.

Clinical appearance: a few hours after drug intake, one or more erythematous or purplish rounded patches appear on the skin and/or on the glans. Lesions can be very swollen and turn into blisters, leading to the development of erosions that heal with a residual hyperpigmentation which increases at each repeated drug exposure. Any cutaneous or mucous site can be affected, but the most frequent localizations are the genitalia and the oral mucosa.

Clinical course: after discontinuing drug intake, the lesions self-heal within a few days, leaving postinflammatory pigmentation. If the same drug is taken again, the lesions relapse and worsen.

Diagnosis: it is based on past medical history and clinical features. In the case of multiple lesions, FDE must be differentiated from erythema multiforme.

Therapy: it consists of discontinuation of the offending drug. Topical corticosteroids and antiseptics are effective in speeding recovery.

Suggested Reading

Baykal Y, Baykal C (2004) Fixed drug eruption of the penis due to zolmitriptan. Dermatology 208:235

Gendernalik SB, Galeckas KJ (2009) Fixed drug eruption: a case report and a review of the literature. Cutis 84:215-9

Lawrentschuk N, Pan D, Troy A (2006) Fixed drug eruption of the penis secondary to sulfamethoxazole-trimethoprim. Scientific World Journal 6:2319-22

Nussinovitch M, Prais D, Ben-Amitai D et al (2002) Fixed drug eruption in the genital area in 15 boys. Pediatr Dermatol 19:216-9

Schuster C, Kränke B, Aberer W, Komericki P (2011) Fixed drug eruption on the penis due to oxcarbazepine. Arch Dermatol 147:362-4

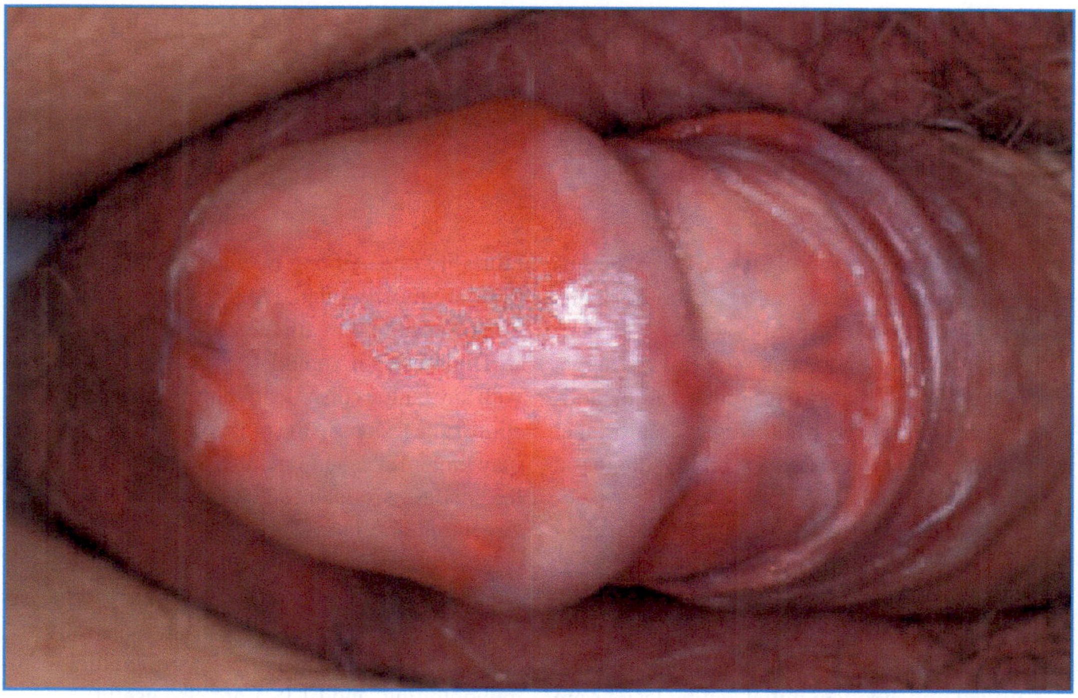

Fig. 5.37 Rounded, glistening, and reddish patch on the glans and foreskin

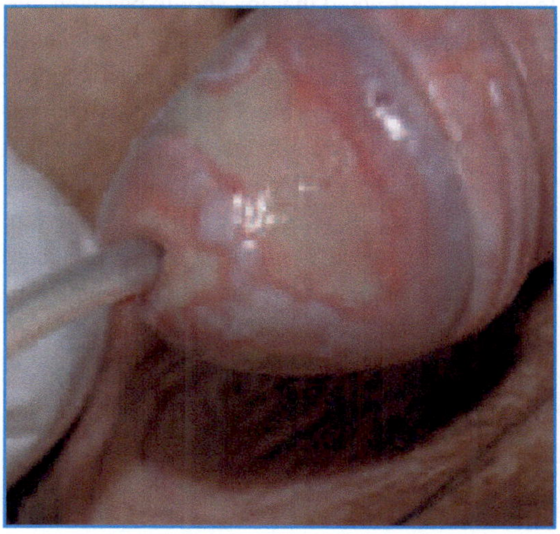

Fig. 5.38 Multiple erosions on the glans

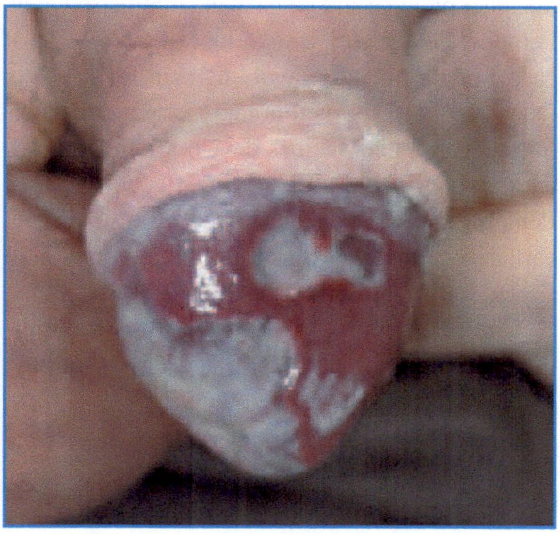

Fig. 5.39 Multiple, confluent, and hemorrhagic erosions of the glans

Pemphigus Vulgaris

Definition: Pemphigus Vulgaris (PV) is an autoimmune, intraepithelial, bullous disorder affecting the skin and mucous membranes.

Etiology: its primary cause is unknown. Its pathogenesis is mediated by circulating autoantibodies directed against keratinocyte desmosomal components (desmogleins) that produce suprabasal acantholysis.

Epidemiology: it affects men and women equally and it is most frequent in middle age. It has been reported to occur worldwide and in all races. Its incidence is about 0.5-3.2 cases per 100,000. Localization in the male genitalia is rare.

Clinical appearance: initial genital lesions are nonspecific superficial erosions located on the glans and prepuce. When the disease progresses, flaccid blisters may occur on the hair-bearing genital area or distant skin. PV can produce scarring of the inner prepuce and glans in uncircumcised men. Pemphigus vegetans is a variant of PV (2-7% of cases) predominantly involving skin folds, scalp, face, and mucous membranes, in which hypertrophic papillated plaques develop in the affected area, obscuring the underlying flaccid blisters. Pemphigus erythematosus represents a superficial variant of pemphigus that implies the formation of flaccid bullae, scaling, erosions and crusting.

Clinical course: PV is a chronic disease requiring lifelong treatment. Untreated PV has a high mortality rate. Among treated patients, complications are mostly related to the side effects of prolonged systemic treatments.

Diagnosis: it should be suspected in patients with any bullous disorder or chronic mucosal ulceration. Like lesions in the oral mucosa, penile lesions may linger for several months or even years before the condition is diagnosed correctly. A biopsy with direct immunofluorescence testing, showing intercellular deposits of IgG or C3 in the epidermis, is mandatory for diagnosis. Indirect immunofluorescence, showing circulating autoantibodies directed against desmoglein-3 or desmoglein-1, immunoblotting, and ELISA are also useful.

Therapy: the most commonly used medications are systemic corticosteroids such as oral prednisone or intravenous methylprednisolone. As PV is a chronic disorder, the onset of side effects from protracted therapy should be taken into consideration. Immunosuppressant agents, such as cyclophosphamide, azathioprine and mycophenolate mofetil, should be considered as steroid-sparing agents. Plasmapheresis can be attempted in refractory cases. Some oral anti-inflammatory antibiotics, such as tetracycline or erythromycin, may be useful in some patients. Local genital care is very important in uncircumcised men with mucous membrane lesions of PV to prevent the development of superinfections and scarring.

Suggested Reading

Palleschi GM, Giomi B, Giacomelli A (2004) Juvenile pemphigus vegetans of the glans penis. Acta Derm Venereol 84:316-7

Sami N, Ahmed AR (2001) Penile pemphigus. Arch Dermatol 137:756-8

Yeh SW, Sami N, Ahmed RA (2005) Treatment of pemphigus vulgaris: current and emerging options. Am J Clin Dermatol 6:327-42

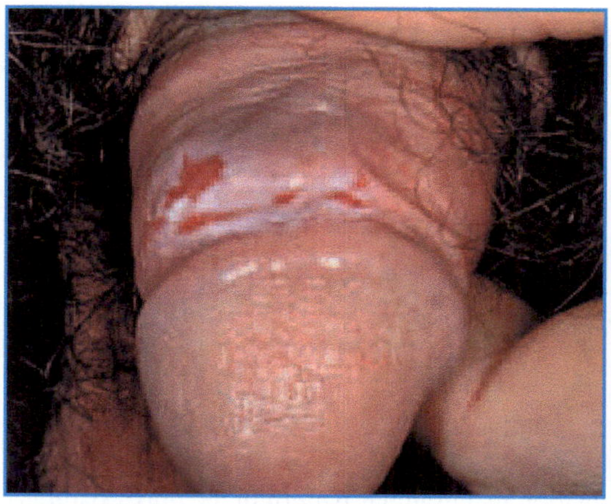

Fig. 5.40 Erosive lesions located on the inner foreskin

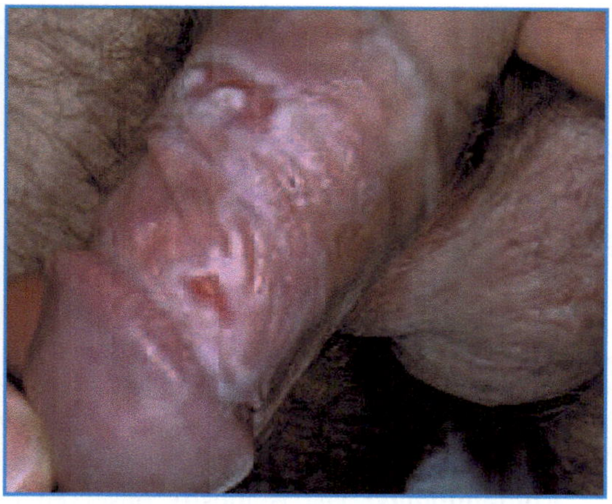

Fig. 5.41 Multiple erosive lesions of the inner foreskin

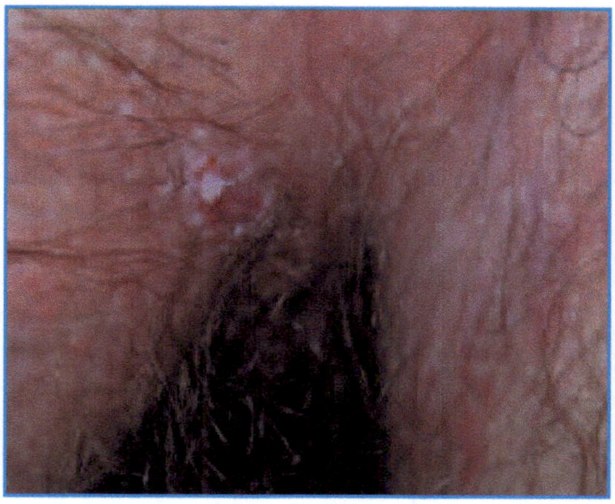

Fig. 5.42 Solitary and erosive lesion on the groin

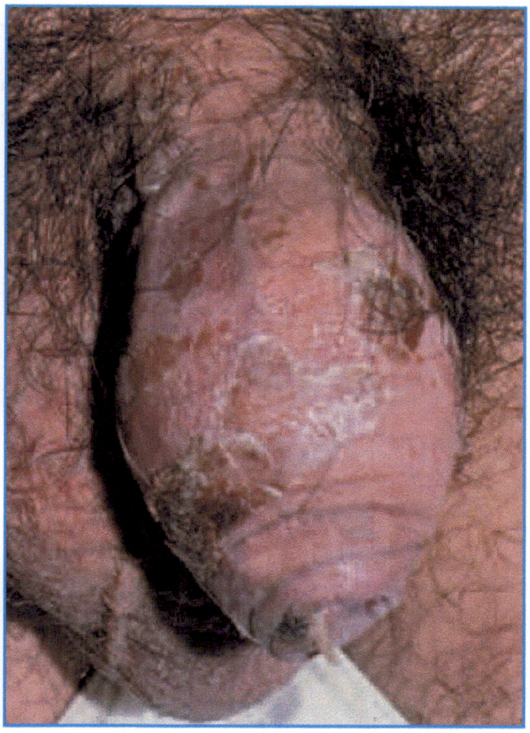

Fig. 5.43 Pemphigus erythematosus: multiple erosions and crusts of the shaft

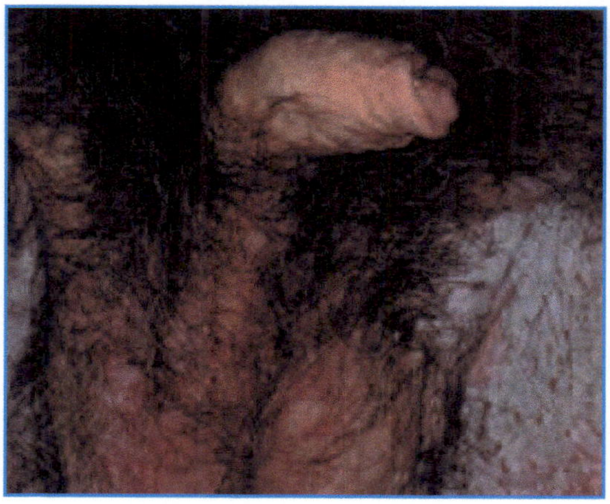

Fig. 5.44 Pemphigus vegetans: grayish and hypertrophic plaques on the groins

Dermatitis Herpetiformis (Dühring's Disease)

Definition: Dermatitis Herpetiformis (DH) is an autoimmune blistering disorder.

Etiology: it is the result of an immunologic response to chronic stimulation of the gut mucosa by dietary gluten.

Epidemiology: DH is mostly observed in young men. Its prevalence has been reported as high as 10 cases per 100,000 population. Among patients with celiac disease, 15-25% develop DH.

Clinical appearance: it is a pruritic condition, initially characterized by erythematous and urticarial plaques, and successively by papules with vesicles and bullae. These lesions may involve the genital area, although other skin areas are usually involved.

Clinical course: DH is a chronic disease. However, it may improve after discontinuing dietary gluten intake.

Diagnosis: it requires direct immunofluorescence of a skin biopsy specimen showing IgA deposition in a granular pattern in the upper papillary dermis. Although most patients are asymptomatic, more than 90% have an associated gluten-sensitive enteropathy upon endoscopic examination.

Therapy: it includes a gluten-free diet and pharmacotherapy. Dapsone (diaminodiphenyl sulfone) and sulfapyridine are the primary medications used to treat DH. Other less effective treatments include colchicine, cyclosporine, azathioprine, and prednisone.

Suggested Reading

Doffoel-Hantz V, Cogné M, Sparsa A et al (2008) Physiopathology of herpetiform dermatitis. Current data. Ann Dermatol Venereol 135:784-8

Fry L (2011) The falling incidence and prevalence of dermatitis herpetiformis. Br J Dermatol 165:229

Rebora A (2011) Shape and configuration of skin lesions: grouped herpetiform. Clin Dermatol 29:509-10

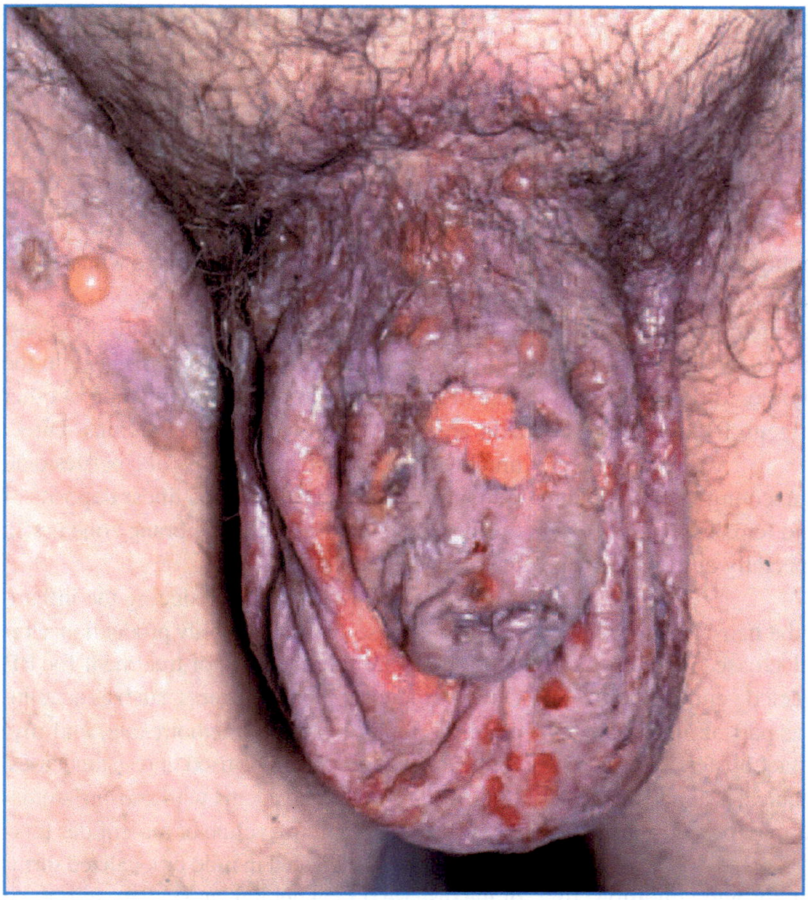

Fig. 5.45 Multiple blisters and erosions in the genital area

Bullous Pemphigoid

Definition: Bullous Pemphigoid (BP) is an autoimmune, subepidermal, blistering disorder that rarely involves the mucous membranes.

Etiology: it is characterized by the presence of circulating IgG autoantibodies directed against the hemidesmosomal antigens BP230 (BPAg1) and BP180 (BPAg2).

Epidemiology: it is an uncommon disease that occurs equally in males and females. It can affect patients at any age, but especially during the sixth to eighth decades of life.

Clinical appearance: the hair-bearing skin of the inner thighs, inguinal crease, scrotum, and perineum are the main affected genital areas. The penis is usually involved as part of a generalized eruption. In such cases, intact blisters are seldom observed and, due to mechanical traumatism, soon develop into erosions that may be asymptomatic and go undiscovered.

Clinical course: it is a chronic condition. Its course is mainly complicated by the side effects of the long-term treatments required, which are a significant concern in elderly patients with several comorbidities.

Diagnosis: genital lesions are more often part of a more generalized form of the disease. In the case of nonspecific findings, examination of other skin areas usually reveals typical lesions. Direct immunofluorescence microscopy of a perilesional skin biopsy that typically shows linear deposits of IgG and/or C3 in the basal membrane zone is still the diagnostic gold standard.

Therapy: it is directed at reducing the inflammatory response and autoantibody production. Corticosteroids are the mainstay of treatment for BP. Other immunosuppressive agents, such as azathioprine, cyclophosphamide, methotrexate, and mycophenolate mofetil, can be used in resistant cases. Dapsone and other oral agents with anti-inflammatory effect, such as tetracycline or macrolides (erythromycin), are indicated in mild or localized forms of the disease. Local genital care is very important in uncircumcised men with mucous membrane lesions because of the risk of infections and scarring.

Suggested Reading

Hertl M, Niedermeier A, Borradori L (2010) Autoimmune bullous skin disorders. Ther Umsch 67:465-82

Ingen-Housz-Oro S, Valeyrie-Allanore L, Ortonne N et al (2011) Management of bullous pemphigoid with topical steroids in the clinical practice of a single center: outcome at 6 and 12 months. Dermatology 222:176-9

Mirza M, Zamilpa I, Wilson JM (2008) Localized penile bullous pemphigoid of childhood. J Pediatr Urol 4:395-7

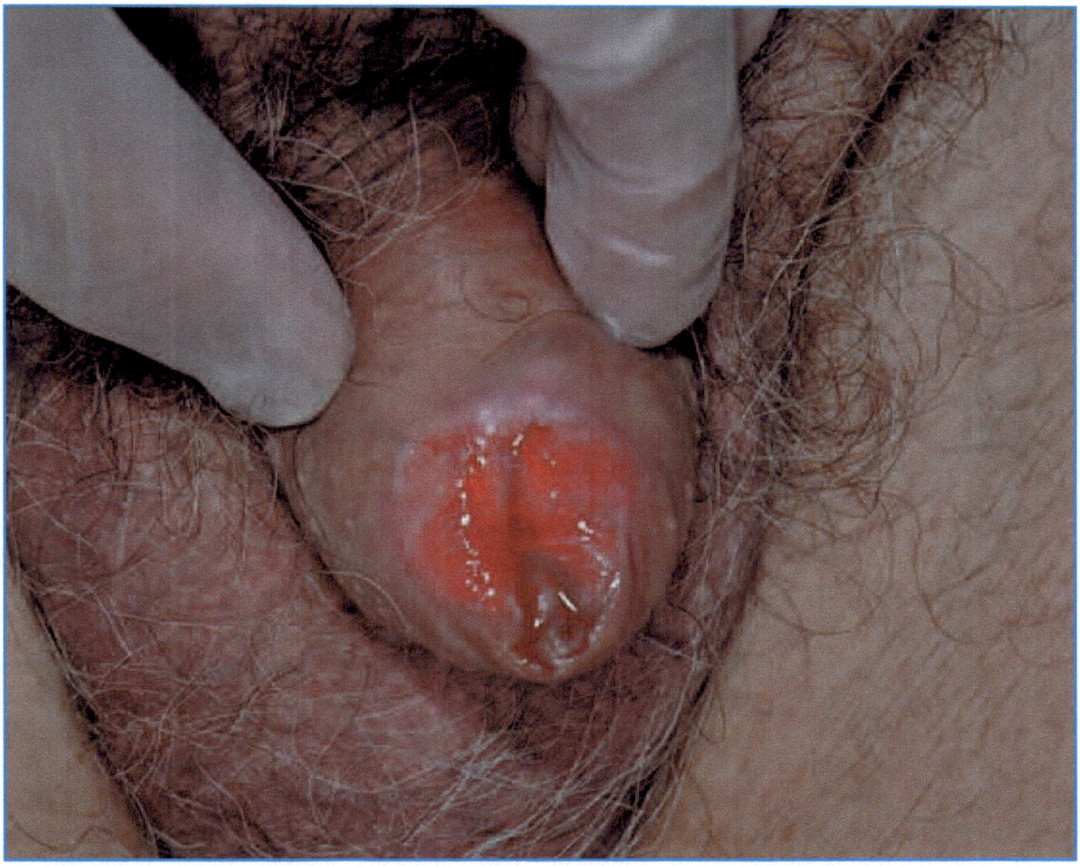

Fig. 5.46 Large, erythematous, and erosive lesion of the foreskin

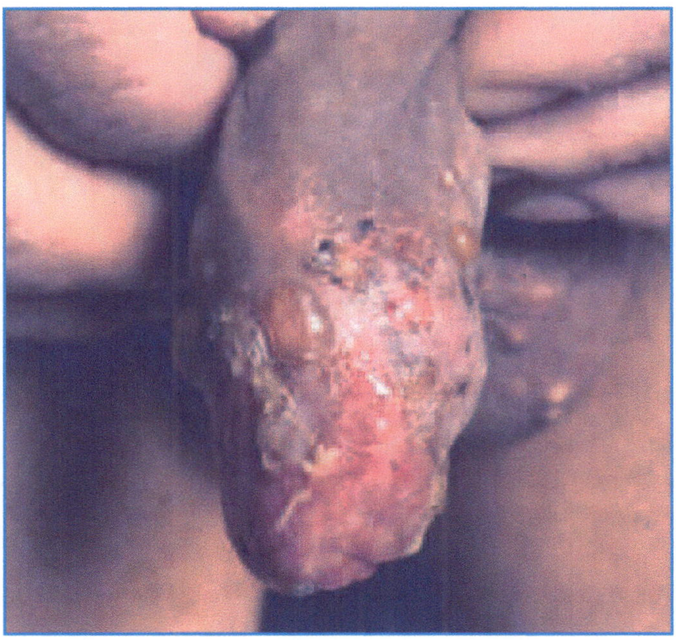

Fig. 5.47 Multiple blisters and erosions of the penis

Hailey-Hailey Disease

Definition: Hailey-Hailey Disease (HHD), also known as benign familial pemphigus, is an inherited bullous skin disorder that predominantly affects the intertriginous areas.

Etiology: ATP2C1, encoding the human secretory pathway Ca(2+)-ATPase (hSPCA1), has been identified as the defective gene of this autosomal dominant disease characterized by abnormal keratinocyte adhesion in the suprabasal layers of the epidermis.

Epidemiology: HHD is a rare condition. It is found worldwide, with a prevalence of approximately 1/50,000. Males and females are equally affected. The symptoms worsen during summer, when the rise in environmental temperature and humidity facilitate superinfections in the intertriginous areas.

Clinical appearance: in the genital area, first small epidermal fragile blisters usually appear in the groin as a result of friction. Subsequently, they evolve into red, eroded, cracked, macerated and foul-smelling plaques. The eruption may also involve the penis and scrotum with similar features.

Clinical course: the disease has an irregular course that depends at least partially on warmth and secondary bacterial and mycotic infections.

Diagnosis: it is usually suggested by the clinical features and the family history. Diagnosis may require a skin biopsy. The histology is characteristic, with layers of detached skin cells ('acantholysis'). Unlike pemphigus vulgaris, in HHD the immunofluorescence test for antibodies is negative.

Therapy: HHD waxes and wanes in intensity. The therapy aims at controlling local environmental precipitating factors and superinfections. Soothing compresses followed by intermittent use of mild corticosteroid preparations and topical antibiotics (clindamycin or erythromycin) result in transient improvement. In resistant cases, systemic dapsone, corticosteroids, methotrexate, retinoids (isotretinoin or acitretin) have been tried with some success.

Suggested Reading

Stolze I, Hamm H, Weyandt GH (2011) Segmental multilayered argon plasma coagulation: effective therapy option for perianal and scrotal Hailey-Hailey disease. Colorectal Dis 13:802-4

Wong TY, Mihm MC Jr (1994) Acantholytic dermatosis localized to genitalia and crural areas of male patients: a report of three cases. J Cutan Pathol 21:27-32

Nasca MR, De Pasquale R, Amodeo S et al (2000) Treatment of Hailey-Hailey disease with oral erythromycin. J Dermatol Treatment 11:273-277

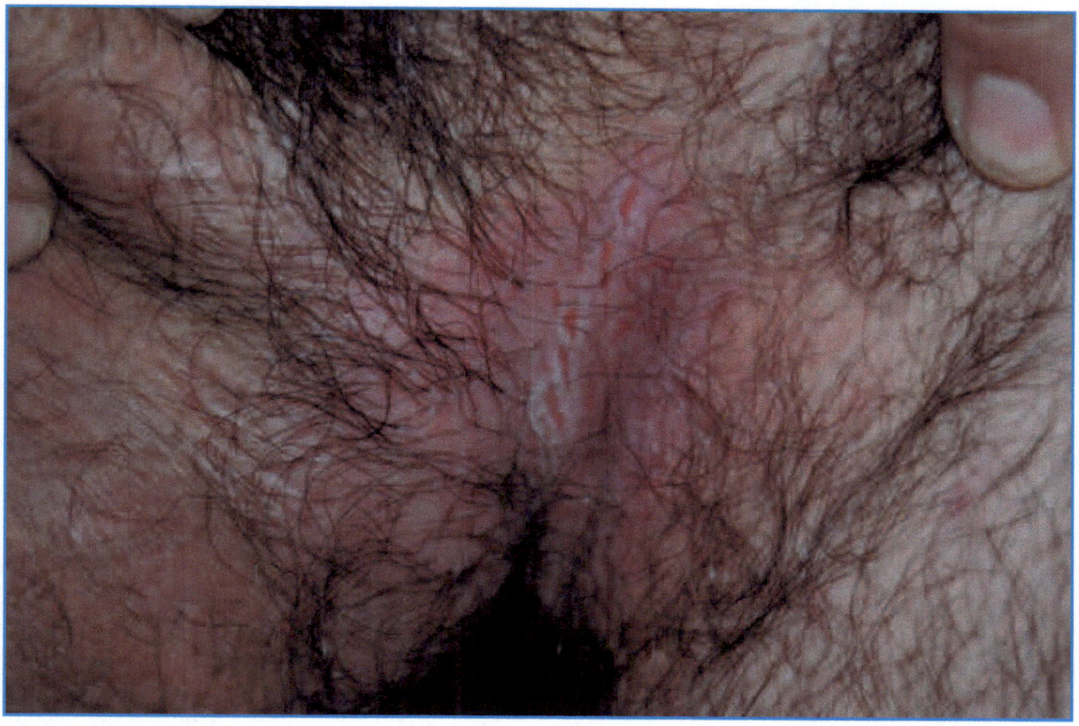

Fig. 5.48 Reddish plaque associated with multiple erosions on the groin

Aphthous Ulcers

Definition: aphthous ulcers, also called aphthae, are benign cutaneous inflammatory lesions that appear and spontaneously heal.

Etiology: it is unknown. It is likely to be multifactorial: genetic, immunological, and psychological factors may contribute to the pathogenesis of the lesions.

Epidemiology: aphthae of the genitalia are not as frequent as those of the oral mucosa. Exact epidemiologic data are not avalaible. They are very rare in men, but are more frequent in women. The peak age of onset is from late childhood to early adulthood.

Clinical appearance: the lesions are often localized on the penis and scrotum, and occasionally on the perianal area. They begin as single, or less often multiple, tiny erythematous macules that soon evolve into small painful ulcers, of size ranging between 0.3 and 2 cm in diameter. They are characteristically sharply marginated and surrounded by an erythematous halo. They are usually round and deep, although larger ones may be irregular in shape.

Clinical course: the lesions usually heal in 2 to 4 weeks, most often without scarring unless they are quite large. The same patient can show oral and genital aphthae, a condition called aphthosis major or bipolar aphthosis. Systemic symptoms, such as fatigue and malaise, can be present in extensive forms of the disease. Frequency of relapses has been reported to gradually decrease after the fifth decade of life.

Diagnosis: the past medical history and the clinical features generally suggest the correct diagnosis. Serologic tests for syphilis, cultures for *H. ducreyii*, and biopsy for malignancy are indicated in equivocal cases. Behçet's syndrome should be excluded if the international diagnostic criteria are not fulfilled.

Therapy: the small asymptomatic lesions can be left untreated. The larger symptomatic ones may require treatment with topical, intralesional or oral corticosteroids. Unresponsive or frequently relapsing cases can be managed by long-term treatment with anti-inflammatory or immunosuppressive agents, such as dapsone, hydroxychloroquine, and azathioprine.

Suggested Reading

Behçet H, Matteson EL (2010) On relapsing, aphthous ulcers of the mouth, eye and genitalia caused by a virus. 1937. Clin Exp Rheumatol 28:S2-5

Liu C, Zhou Z, Liu G et al (2012) Efficacy and safety of dexamethasone ointment on recurrent aphthous ulceration. Am J Med 125:292-301

O'Neill ID (2012) Efficacy of tumour necrosis factor-α antagonists in aphthous ulceration: review of published individual patient data. J Eur Acad Dermatol Venereol 26:231-5

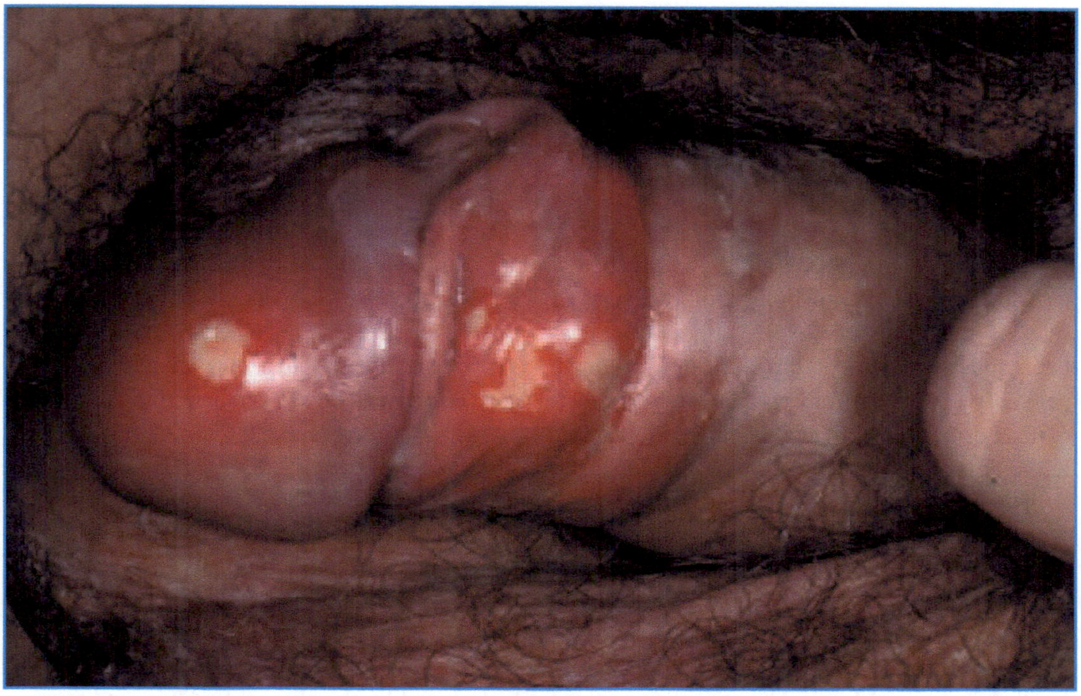

Fig. 5.49 Typical small and "punched out" lesions involving the glans and the inner foreskin

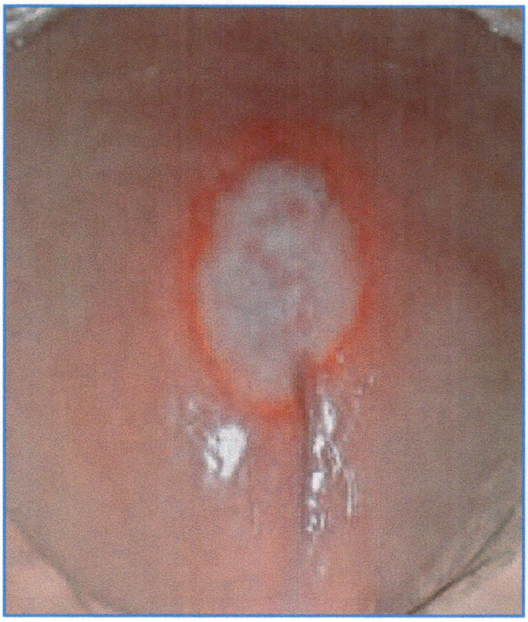

Fig. 5.50 Large lesion of the glans

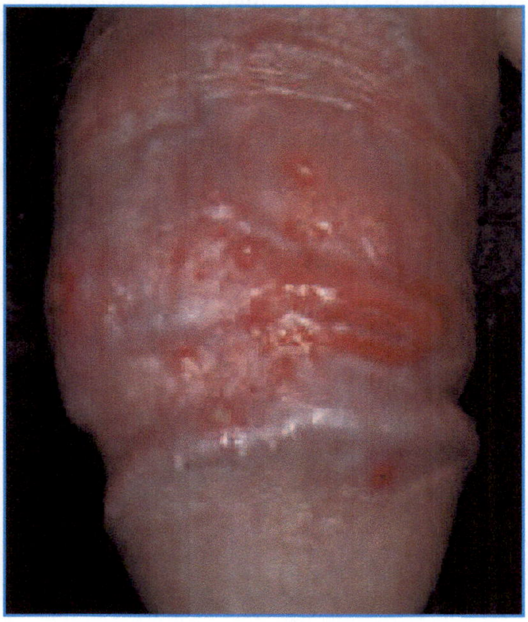

Fig. 5.51 Multiple, small, and herpes-like lesions on the glans

Behçet's Disease

Definition: Behçet's disease (BD) is a systemic necrotising vasculitis affecting blood vessels of all sizes. It is characterized by oral aphthae in all patients and by at least 2 of the following symptoms: genital aphthae, cutaneous pustular vasculitis, synovitis, posterior uveitis, and meningoencephalitis, in the absence of inflammatory bowel disease or collagen-vascular disease.

Etiology: it is unknown, but a pathogenic role of Th1-mediated immune response has been suggested. Pathergy, i.e., the development of skin lesions after trauma or injury, may occur.

Epidemiology: BD is described in Europe, North America and Japan. The variant recognized in Western Europe and North America includes oral and genital ulceration and it is less severe. "Western" BD is more frequent in female patients and often presents as collagen-vascular disease. "Eastern" BD is more frequent in male patients and often presents as a central nervous system and ocular disorder.

Clinical appearance: the lesions, generally superficial, appear as "punched out" small ulcers and are extremely painful and tender. Genital ulcers occur in about 90% of patients, and generally recur in crops (many shallow ulcers at the same time). They range in size from a few mm to 2 cm in diameter. They usually occur on the scrotum, less often on the penis, and can heal with residual scarring.

Clinical course: the disease relapses into acute episodes for many years. In addition to the mucosal ulcers, patients can present diarrhea, arthritis, thrombophlebitis, and psychiatric and neurologic problems. In severe cases, BD can lead to blindness, meningoencephalitis or stroke.

Diagnosis: it is supported by the past medical history and by the clinical findings, and requires fulfilment of the international diagnostic criteria (see definition).

Therapy: first-line therapies include topical or intralesional corticosteroids and topical tacrolimus. Dapsone and colchicine may be beneficial for some patients. Since high serum levels of TNF and soluble TNF receptors have been found in BD, therapy with TNF blockers is an option to consider when other therapies fail.

Suggested Reading

Davatchi F, Shahram F, Chams-Davatchi C et al (2010) Behçet's disease: from East to West. Clin Rheumatol 29:823-33
Dilsen N (1996) History and development of Behçet's disease. Rev Rhum Engl Ed 63:512-9
Mendes D, Correia M, Barbedo M et al (2009) Behçet's disease—a contemporary review. J Autoimmun 32:178-88
Yesudian PD, Edirisinghe DN, O'Mahony C (2007) Behçet's disease. Int J STD AIDS 18:221-7

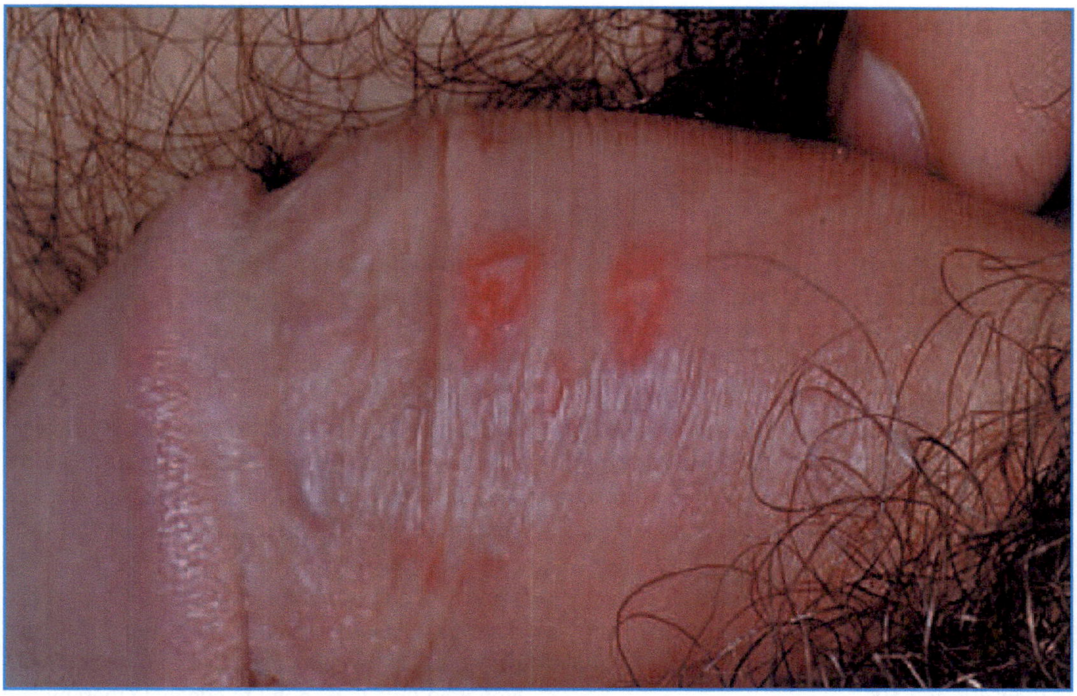

Fig. 5.52 Aphthous ulcers on the shaft

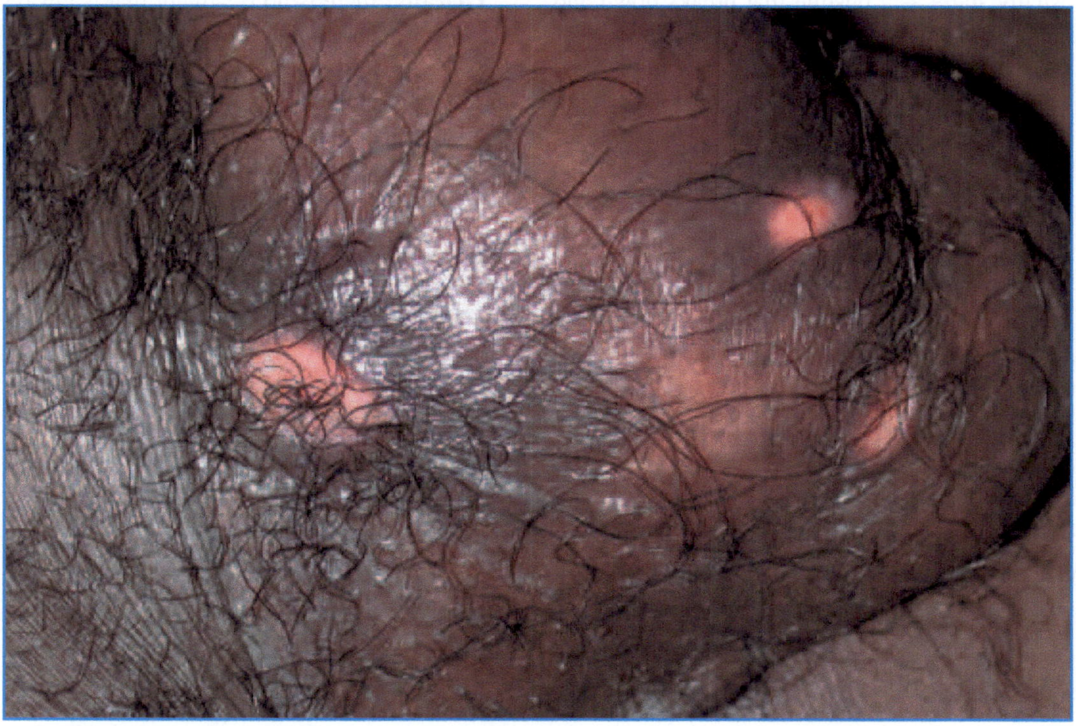

Fig. 5.53 Multiple aphthous ulcers on the scrotum in an Afro-American patient

Pyoderma Gangrenosum

Definition: Pyoderma Gangrenosum (PG) is a destructive, neutrophilic inflammatory disorder, mostly involving the lower extremities, which can also involve the hands, head, neck, and genitals.

Etiology: it is not well understood, but the disease is thought to be due to immune system dysregulation, and particularly to neutrophil dysfunction. Ulcerations of PG may occur after skin trauma or injury in 30% of patients; this process is called *pathergy*.

Epidemiology: it is a rare disease. Its annual incidence in the United States is approximately 1 case per 100,000 people. It mostly affects people in their 40s and 50s.

Clinical appearance: different clinical manifestations have been described, including ulcerative, pustular, bullous, and vegetative variants. PG usually starts as a pustule that breaks down and turns into an enlarging ulcer, usually with a typical violaceous, frequently raised, undermined border. Ulcers can be single or multiple. The genital location in men is very rare.

Clinical course: it may occur alone even though, in about 50% of patients, PG is associated with an underlying systemic disease, such as inflammatory bowel disease, arthritis, and hematologic malignancy.

Diagnosis: it is one of exclusion, with penile lesions having a substantial differential diagnosis from infections like syphilis, herpes simplex, mycobacterial ulceration, and amoebiasis, and from noninfectious causes of genital ulceration like squamous cell carcinoma, cutaneous Crohn's disease, and ulcerating sarcoidosis. PG should be suspected in any patient with an ulcerative penile lesion who fails to respond to adequate therapy and who has a negative or nonconfirmatory diagnostic evaluation for infectious or other inflammatory conditions.

Therapy: there is no treatment that is always effective. The most consistent results are reported with systemic corticosteroids and cyclosporine. Topical tacrolimus and imiquimod represent interesting novel approaches to treatment. Effective management of an underlying disorder often seems to result in improvement of the PG.

Suggested Reading

Das NK, Dutta RN (2010) Pyoderma gangrenosum on glans penis: an unusual site. J Indian Med Assoc 108:873-4

Georgala S, Georgala C, Nicolaidou E (2008) Pyoderma gangrenosum of the penis: a potentially dramatic skin disease. Urology 72:1185

Kim TH, Oh SY, Myung SC (2009) Pyoderma gangranosum of the penis. J Korean Med Sci 24:1200-2

Parren LJ, Nellen RG, Van Marion AM et al (2008) Penile pyoderma gangrenosum: successful treatment with colchicine. Int J Dermatol 47:7-9

Crohn's Disease

Definition: Crohn's Disease (CD) is an inflammatory granulomatous disease that may affect any part of the gastrointestinal tract from mouth to anus, causing a wide variety of symptoms. It can directly affect the skin of the involved bowel (contiguous form), or it can affect sites distant from the gastrointestinal tract (noncontiguous form); this phenomenon is also known as "metastatic CD".

Etiology: it is unknown. It is believed that CD is caused by interactions between environmental, immunological and bacterial factors in genetically susceptible individuals. This results in a chronic inflammatory disorder, possibly directed to microbial antigens, in which the host immune system attacks the gastrointestinal tract. Psychological factors may be triggers for the periodic exacerbations of the disease.

Epidemiology: there is a paucity of literature describing the occurrence of genital CD in men. Although perianal involvement occurs in nearly one-third of patients with CD and cutaneous involvement can be seen in 22-44%, genital manifestations are extremely rare. CD typically presents after the onset of bowel symptoms, although it has been reported to precede bowel symptoms by 3 months to 8 years in 20% of patients.

Clinical appearance: genital CD can present in several different forms. It can occur as a result of direct extension from areas near the bowel, such as the anus or a colostomy site, or it can appear on the genitalia as a solitary lesion. Male and female genital lesions usually appear as a nonhealing ulcer, but they can present as a papule, a plaque, or swelling. Penile and scrotal edema may occur. Linear fissures can develop within intertriginous folds. This sign, termed "knife cut", is a very distinctive finding. Interestingly, the severity of the cutaneous findings may not correlate with the severity of the bowel symptoms.

Clinical course: the anogenital disease persists for long periods of time with little evidence of spontaneous remission. Healing of anogenital lesions usually occurs with scarring. CD can cause abdominal pain, diarrhea, vomiting, or weight loss, but it may also give rise to extraintestinal manifestations with cutaneous involvement.

Diagnosis: diagnosis of noncontiguous genital CD is based on clinical history and histological findings, showing in the dermis the typical non-caseating granulomas arranged in a perivascular distribution.

Therapy: there is no specific treatment for genital involvement of Crohn's disease. Topical and systemic corticosteroids, sulfasalazine, azathioprine, metronidazole, tetracyclines, dapsone, and hyperbaric oxygen, have been used with success. A few cases in which circumcision was required have been described. Recently, the efficacy of combined treatment with topical tacrolimus and systemic prednisone has been reported.

Suggested Reading

Lane VA, Vajda P, King D et al (2010) Metastatic Crohn's disease: two cases of penile Crohn's and literature review. J Pediatr Urol 6:270-3

Lopez V, Alonso V, Monteagudo C et al (2009) Penile and scrotal edema as a manifestation of Crohn's disease. Int J Dermatol 48:1136-7

Rajpara S, Siddha S, Ormerod A et al (2008) Cutaneous penile and perianal Crohn's disease treated with a combination of medical and surgical interventions. Aust J Dermatol 49:21-24

Reyes M, Borum M (2009) Severe case of genital and perianal cutaneous Crohn's disease. Inflamm Bowel Dis 15:1125-6

Lichen Sclerosus

Definition: Lichen Sclerosus (LS) is a chronic inflammatory disease that affects the genitalia and less often the extragenital skin (upper trunk and arms).

Etiology: although uncertain, the etiology seems to be multifactorial, including genetic, autoimmune, and hormonal factors.

Epidemiology: it can occur in patients of any age group, sex, or race, but seems to be more common in prepuberal girls and postmenopausal women. It is most common in whites and rare in blacks. About 10% of male patients with genital LS present extragenital locations. The exact prevalence is unknown, but estimates range from 1:60 to 1:1,000.

Clinical appearance: anal and scrotal involvement is rare and the lesions are generally localized on penile skin and mucosa. LS occurs on the glans and foreskin as erythematous papules and plaques that rapidly become whitish and hard in consistency. The skin and the mucosa slowly become atrophic and this fragility may lead to the development of erosions and purpura, and less commonly to hemorrhagic blistering. As the disease progresses, scarring may cause the formation of synechiae and phimosis. Itching and burning are common symptoms.

Clinical course: prepuberal LS is generally self-healing, while adult LS has a chronic course. If not treated, in men LS can lead to various complications such as preputial adhesion, phimosis, paraphimosis, and urethral stenosis. Moreover, LS is associated with a higher risk of developing a squamous cell carcinoma in the genital area, while malignancies have not been reported in extragenital regions. LS generates discomfort and incapacity for sexual intercourse.

Diagnosis: the clinical features are usually diagnostic but in doubtful cases, or to rule out malignancy, a histopatological examination must be performed. Depending on the clinical findings, the differential diagnosis may include erosive lichen planus, lichen simplex, leukoplakia, and vitiligo.

Therapy: it is aimed at reducing pain and the burning sensation, at healing the mucocutaneous lesions, and at preventing permanent scarring and the development of malignancies. First-line treatment includes topical therapy with corticosteroids and calcineurin-inhibitors. If the therapy is protracted, the risk of bacterial, mycotic, and viral superinfections should be taken into account, prompting specific treatment in case such complications should occur. Other treatments, such as topical testosterone and calcipotriol, cryosurgery, phototherapy and photodynamic therapy, have been proposed, but none has proved to be more effective than topical corticosteroids. Circumcision can produce improvement in adult men and resolution in young men. Urethral stenosis may require surgical therapy. Careful follow-up is recommended for timely detection and treatment of incipient squamous cell carcinoma.

Suggested Reading

Clouston D, Hall A, Lawrentschuk N (2011) Penile lichen sclerosus (balanitis xerotica obliterans). BJU Int 108:14-9

Edmonds EV, Hunt S, Hawkins D et al (2012) Clinical parameters in male genital lichen sclerosus: a case series of 329 patients. J Eur Acad Dermatol Venereol 26:730-7

Garaffa G, Shabbir M, Christopher N et al (2011) The surgical management of lichen sclerosus of the glans penis: our experience and review of the literature. J Sex Med 8:1246-53

Innocenzi D, Nasca MR, Skroza N et al (2006) Penile lichen sclerosus: Correlation between histopathologic features and risk of cancer. Acta Dermatovenerol Croat 14:225-9

Nasca MR, Innocenzi D, Micali G (1999) Penile cancer among patients with genital lichen sclerosus. J Am Acad Dermatol 41:911-4

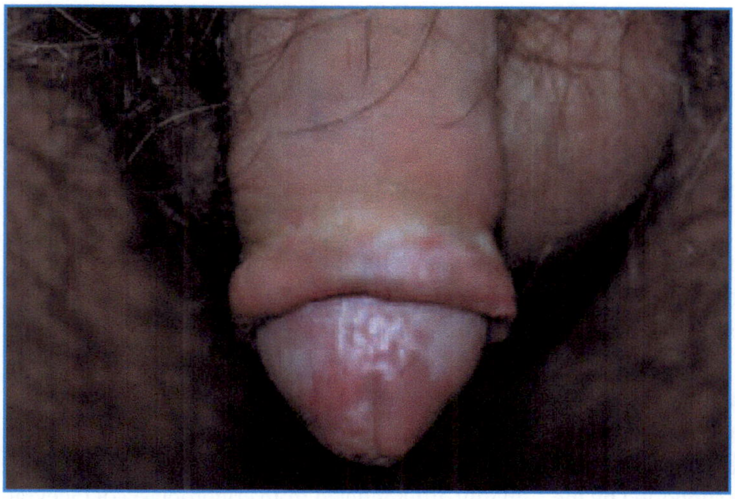

Fig. 5.54 Erythematous and whitish sclerotic plaques of the glans and foreskin

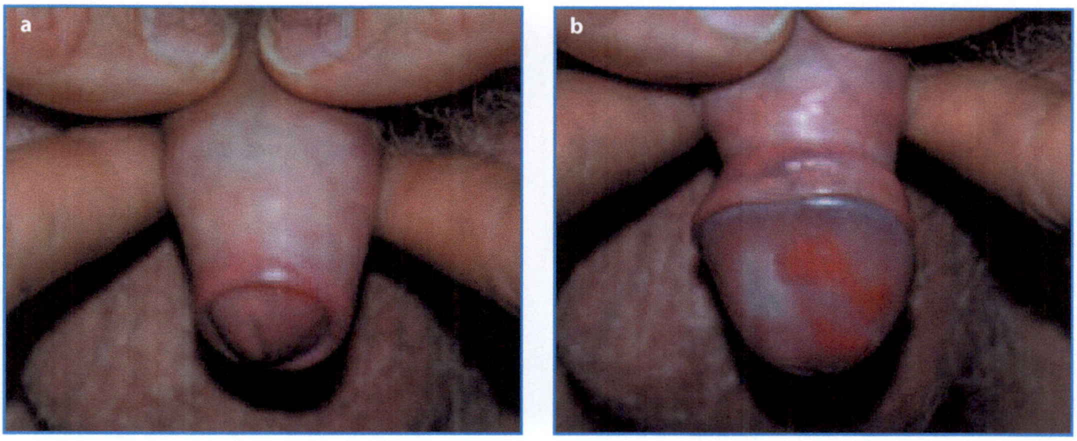

Fig. 5.55 a Sclerosis of the foreskin. **b** Whitish plaques and erosive lesions of the glans

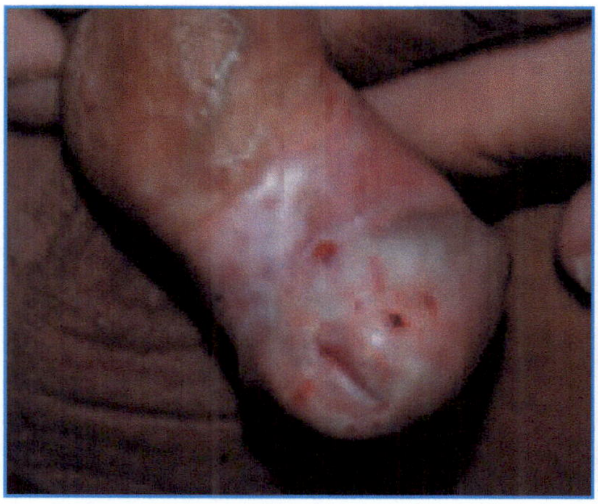

Fig. 5.56 Whitish, coalescent sclerotic plaques, synechiae, and hemorrhagic lesions of the glans and foreskin

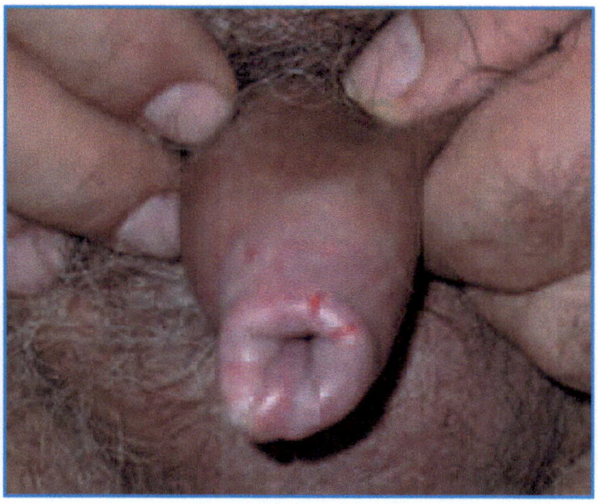

Fig. 5.57 Phimosis and fissuring of the foreskin

Plasma Cell Balanitis (Zoon)

Definition: Plasma Cell Balanitis (PCB), also known as Zoon balanitis, is an inflammatory disease with chronic-relapsing course and benign behaviour.

Etiology: it is not well known, the friction between the glans and the prepuce and related microbiological alterations are believed to play an important role. This consideration is supported by the absence of the condition in circumcised men.

Epidemiology: it is a common disease in middle-aged and older uncircumcised men. It is unusual in young people.

Clinical appearances: it is characterized by a single erythematous, or erythematous-brownish, sharply marginated patch on the glans and/or the inner foreskin, 1.5 cm or more in diameter, with a bright, smooth, and sometimes erosive surface. It is usually asymptomatic.

Clinical course: it is chronic with continual relapses.

Diagnosis: the clinical features can suggest the diagnosis but, in many cases, histopathological confirmation is necessary. This condition must be primarily differentiated from erythroplasia of Queyrat, which may often clinically resemble PCB.

Therapy: topical corticosteroids and calcineurin inhibitors (tacrolimus and pimecrolimus) are effective, but the recurrence rate is very high, while circumcision can be a definitive treatment. Some authors have reported the efficacy of CO_2 laser therapy.

Suggested Reading

Kumar B, Narang T, Dass Radotra B, Gupta S (2006) Plasma cell balanitis: clinicopathologic study of 112 cases and treatment modalities. J Cutan Med Surg 10:11-5

Nasca MR, De Pasquale R, Micali G (2007) Treatment of Zoon's balanitis with imiquimod 5% cream. J Drugs Dermatol 6:532-4

Pastar Z, Rados J, Lipozenci J et al (2004) Zoon plasma cell balanitis: an overview and role of histopathology. Acta Dermatovenerol Croat 12:268-73

Retamar RA, Kien MC, Chouela EN (2003) Zoon's balanitis: presentation of 15 patients, five treated with a carbon dioxide laser. Int J Dermatol 42:305-7

Weyers W, Ende Y, Schalla W, Diaz-Cascajo C (2002) Balanitis of Zoon: a clinicopathologic study of 45 cases. Am J Dermatopathol 24:459-67

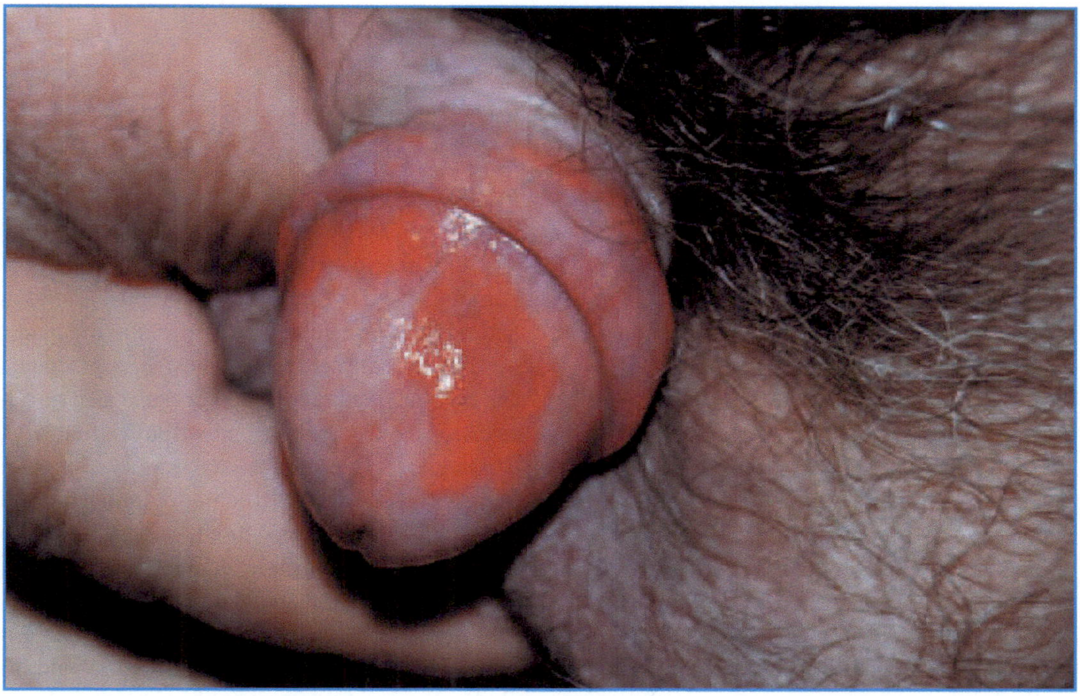

Fig. 5.58 Sharply demarcated, glistening, and red patches on the glans

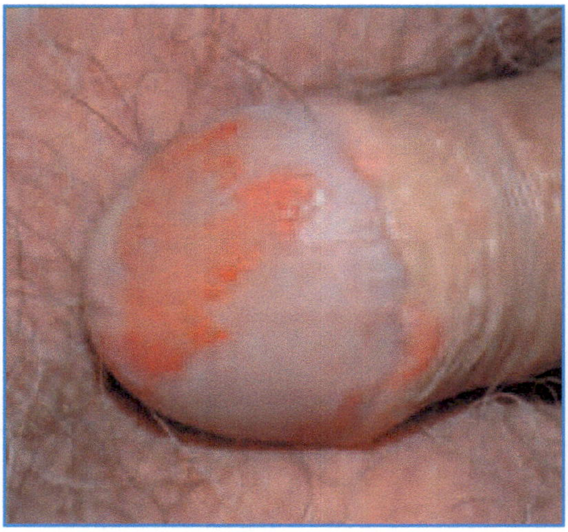

Fig. 5.59 Smooth, confluent, and erythematous patches on the glans and foreskin

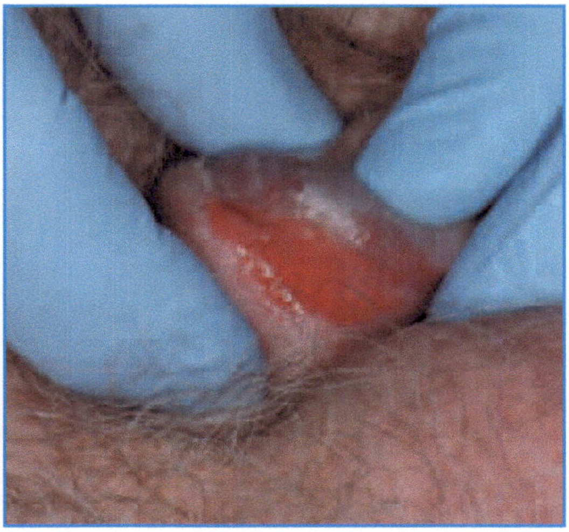

Fig. 5.60 Glistening and red patches on the foreskin

Angioedema

Definition: angioedema is an acute, inflammatory disorder characterized by the rapid onset of edema involving cutaneous, subcutaneous, and mucosal tissues.

Etiology: it can be caused by a localized allergic reaction. Consequently, it may occur in association with other allergic symptoms, such as urticaria. Genital involvement is more often reported in subjects with latex allergy (condoms or diaphrams) or sensitized to their partner's genital discharge. An inherited autosomal dominant variant resulting from a deficiency or a dysfunction of the C1 inhibitor, localized in the gastrointestinal and upper respiratory tracts, without signs or symptoms of urticaria, is also well known.

Epidemiology: genital angioedema is a rare condition.

Clinical appearance: it is characterized by recurrent episodes of edema involving both skin and mucosa of genital area, especially the glans.

Clinical course: when extensive, angioedema can be a medical emergency because airway obstruction can occur, leading to asphyxiation.

Diagnosis: it is clinical. Laboratory investigations for C4, C1q, and C1 inhibitor (antigenic and functional) blood levels should be performed to rule out hereditary angioedema. Testing for allergy is also recommended.

Therapy: the treatment of idiopathic angioedema is the same as that of urticaria, and includes the use of systemic antihistamines and corticosteroids. Hereditary angioedema requires proper prophylactic strategies and pharmacological management of acute attacks.

Suggested Reading

Banerji A (2010) Current treatment of hereditary angioedema: An update on clinical studies. Allergy Asthma Proc 1:398-406

Dhairyawan R, Harrison R, Buckland M, Hourihan M (2011) Hereditary angioedema: an unusual cause of genital swelling presenting to a genitourinary medicine clinic. Int J STD AIDS 22:356-7

Johnston DT (2011) Diagnosis and management of hereditary angioedema. J Am Osteopath Assoc 111:28-36

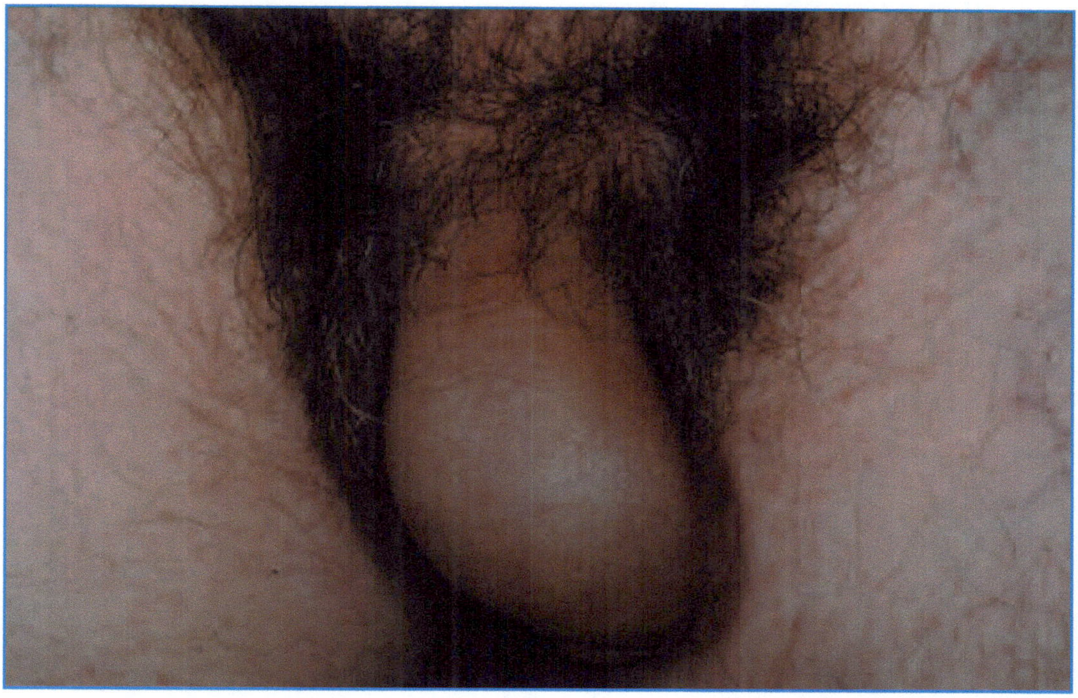

Fig. 5.61 Penile edema due to latex allergy

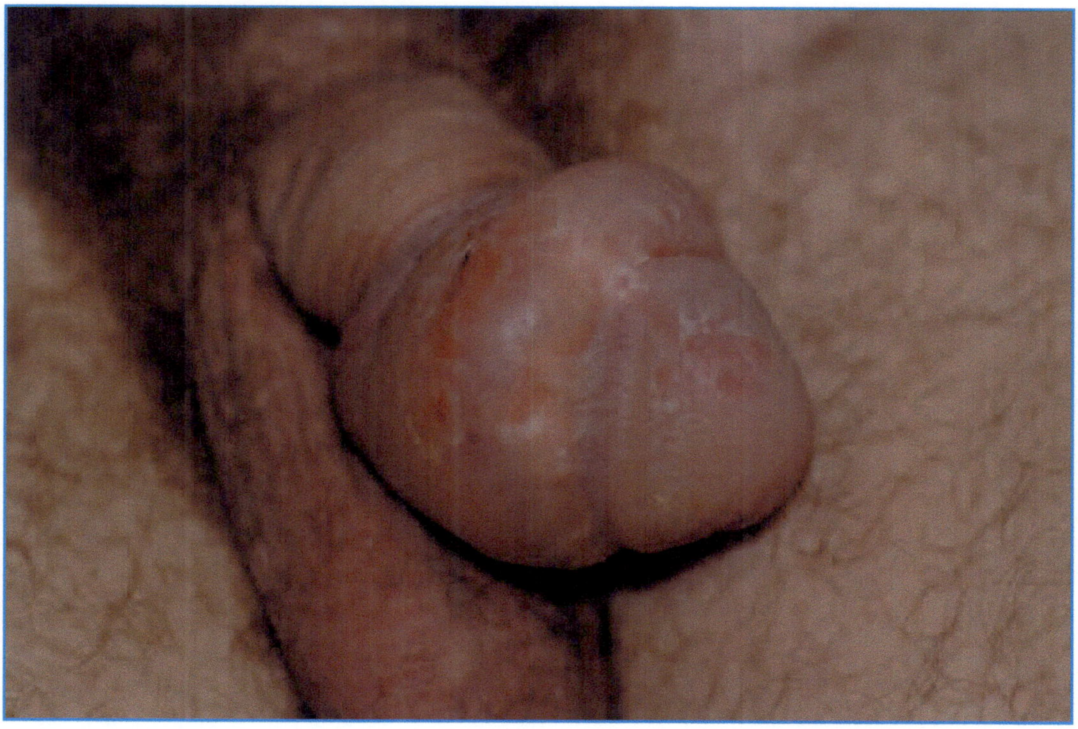

Fig. 5.62 Marked edema of the foreskin

6 Pigmentation Disorders

Pompeo Donofrio, Paola Donofrio,
Maria Grazia Francia, and Giuseppe Micali

P. Donofrio (✉)
School of Dermatology and Venereology
"Federico II" University of Naples, Naples, Italy
e-mail: dermodonofrio@hotmail.it

G. Micali et al., *Atlas of Male Genital Disorders*,
DOI: 10.1007/978-88-470-2787-9_6, © Springer-Verlag Italia 2013

Vitiligo

Definition: vitiligo is an acquired pigmentary disorder of the skin and mucous membranes, characterized by circumscribed hypopigmented macules and patches.

Etiology: it is a multifactorial polygenic disorder with a complex pathogenesis, related both to genetic and nongenetic factors. The autoimmune theory hypothesises an alteration in humoral and cellular immunity, which causes melanocyte damage. Thyroid disorders (Hashimoto thyroiditis and Graves' disease), endocrinopathies such as Addison's disease and diabetes mellitus, alopecia areata, pernicious anemia, inflammatory bowel disease, psoriasis, and autoimmune polyglandular syndrome are commonly associated with vitiligo.

Epidemiology: vitiligo affects 0.5-2% of the world population; the average age of onset is 20 years.

Clinical appearance: the most common form of vitiligo is an amelanotic macule or patch of variable size. The lesions may be multiple and confluent. They are usually roundish, with sharp convex borders, chalky white, and centrifugally enlarging. The genitalia are a common site for depigmentation, and vitiligo may often impair the psychosexual function of affected men.

Clinical course: it is a benign disorder with a chronic relapsing course.

Diagnosis: it is generally made on the basis of clinical findings. Wood's lamp examination may be useful. Biopsy is occasionally helpful for differentiating vitiligo from other hypopigmentary disorders.

Therapy: the treatment of vitiligo is troublesome. Topical or systemic corticosteroids, topical calcineurin inhibitors, and phototherapy are among the most popular therapies, but UV radiation should be avoided for the treatment of genital area, because of the risk of squamous cell carcinoma development. It is well recognized that the response to treatment may be considerably different among different patients and, in the same patient, it may depend on the anatomic location of the lesions. Treatment must be tailored, and patients should be made aware of the risks associated with therapy.

Suggested Reading

Bhandarkar SS, Kundu RV (2012) Quality-of-life issues in vitiligo. Dermatol Clin 30:255-68

Bulat V, Situm M, Dediol I et al (2011) The mechanisms of action of phototherapy in the treatment of the most common dermatoses. Coll Antropol 35:147-51

Miniati A, Weng Z, Zhang B et al (2012) Neuro-immuno-endocrine processes in vitiligo pathogenesis. Int J Immunopathol Pharmacol 25:1-7

Patel NS, Paghdal KV, Cohen GF (2012) Advanced treatment modalities for vitiligo. Dermatol Surg 38:381-91

Picardo M (2012) Vitiligo: new insights. Br J Dermatol 166:472-3

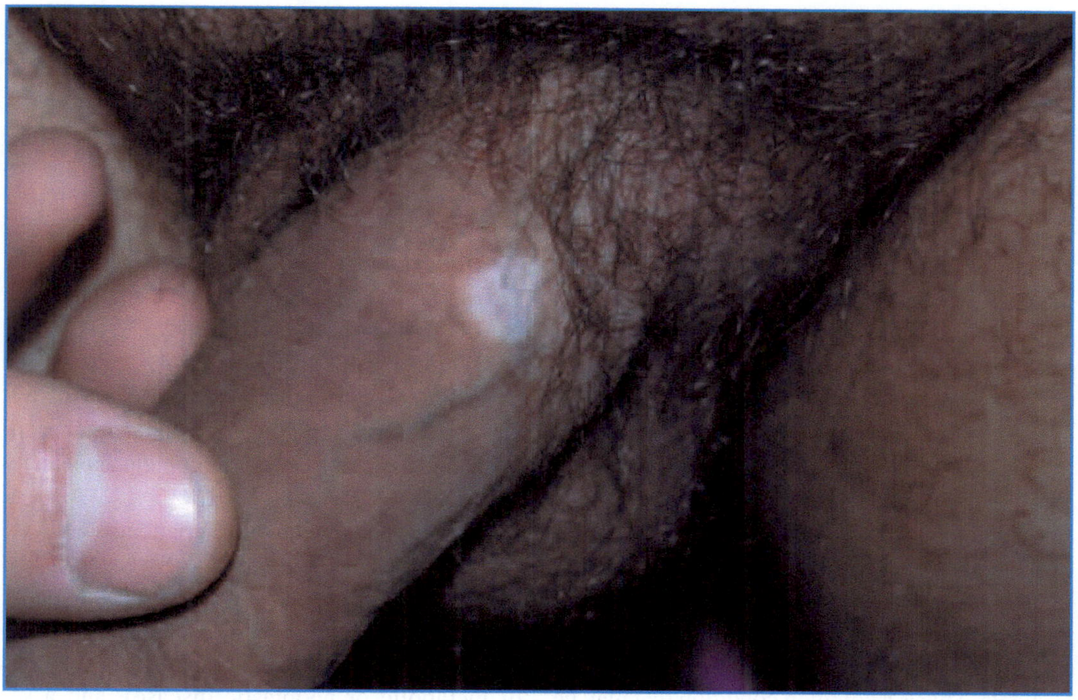

Fig. 6.1 Solitary, round, and white patch on the proximal shaft

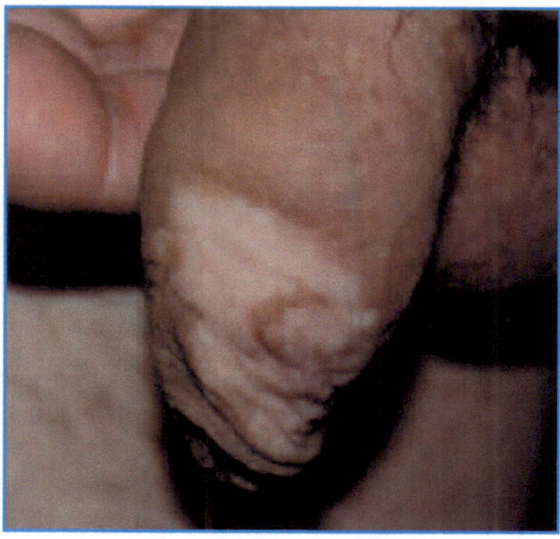

Fig. 6.2 White and sharply marginated patch involving the shaft and the foreskin

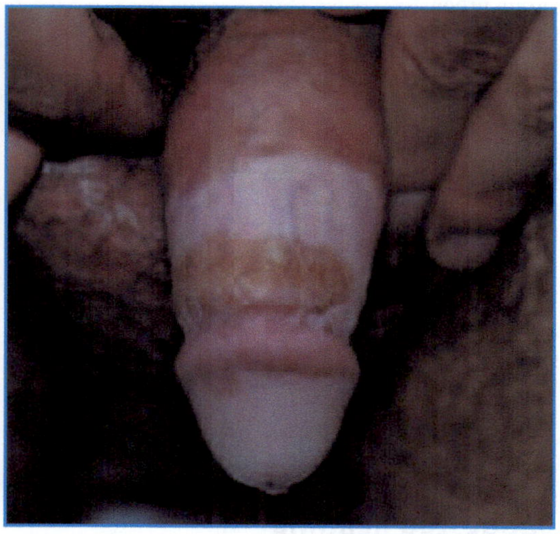

Fig. 6.3 White and confluent patches involving the glans, the foreskin, and the shaft

Acanthosis Nigricans

Definition: Acanthosis Nigricans (AN) is a pigmented disorder of the skin.

Etiology: it is not yet known. Hyperinsulinemia (with or without diabetes mellitus), hyperandrogenemia (with or without virilism), metabolic disorders, drugs (nicotinic acid, corticosteroids, estrogens, insulin, fusidic acid, protease inhibitors, recombinant growth hormone), and malignancy (most commonly gastric adenocarcinoma, less frequently endocrine, genitourinary and lung carcinomas, melanoma) have been suggested as causative factors.

Epidemiology: no reliable data are currently available. This is a common condition that may be underdiagnosed.

Clinical appearance: AN is clinically characterized by hyperpigmented, verrucous or velvety plaques, usually present on flexural and intertriginous areas.

Clinical course: it is a benign condition in itself, although some cases may be associated with an underlying visceral malignancy.

Diagnosis: it is generally easily made on the basis of clinical findings. Histology, showing hyperkeratosis and papillomatosis, but neither acanthosis nor increased melanin content, is usually unnecessary.

Therapy: management of patients with AN can be quite challenging. The first step is the identification of the underlying cause, which generally requires an accurate medical history, a complete medical examination (searching for the signs of metabolic or neoplastic disease), and a selected panel of laboratory tests. In most cases, the treatment of the underlying disease clears up the cutaneous disorder.

Suggested Reading

Dubnov-Raz G, Weiss R, Raz R et al (2011) Acanthosis nigricans and truncal fat in overweight and obese children. J Pediatr Endocrinol Metab 24:697-701

Kumar KV, Priya S, Shaikh A, Prusty P (2011) Diabetes in young unusual case presentation. J Pediatr Endocrinol Metab 24:581-3

Sehgal VN, Srivastava G, Aggarwal AK et al (2011) Noninsulin-dependent, type II diabetes mellitus-related dermatoses: part II. Skinmed 9:302-8

Valdés Rodríguez R, Moncada González B, Rivera Rodríguez SP et al (2011) Skin tags and Acanthosis nigricans: association with insulin resistance and overweight in Mexican children. Gac Med Mex 147:297-302

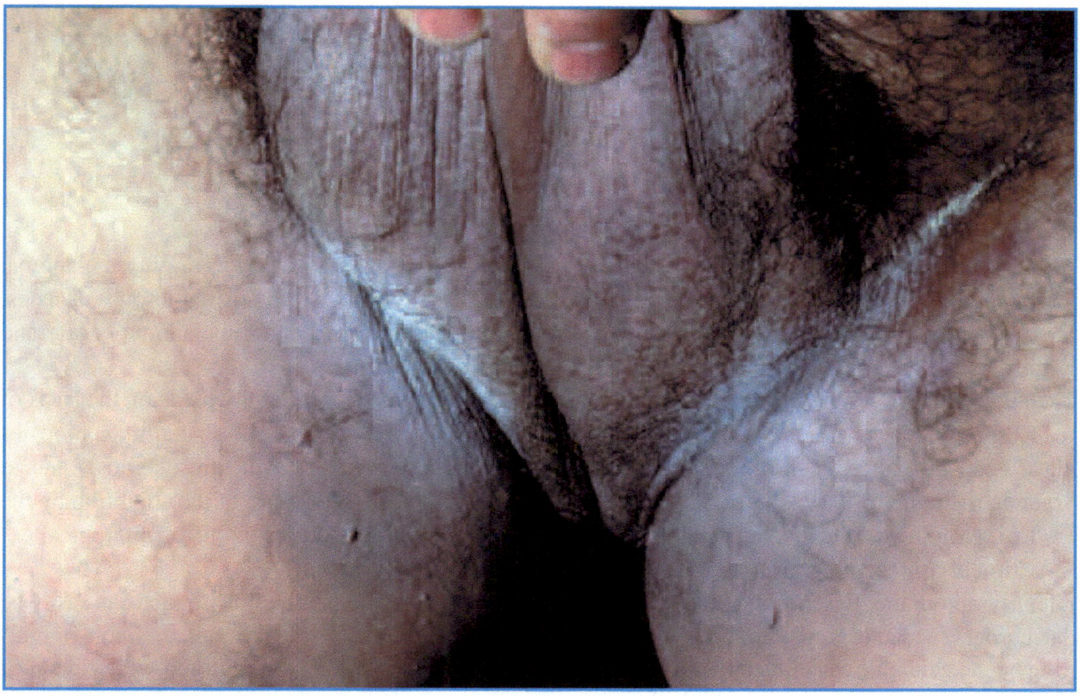

Fig. 6.4 Hyperpigmented and velvety inguinal plaques

Melanosis

Definition: melanosis (lentiginosis) is a benign pigmented lesion of mucosa and skin characterized by pigmentation of basal keratinocytes with normal, or a slightly increased number of, melanocytes.

Etiology: it is considered idiopathic, but cases have been described in the literature related to trauma, irritation or PUVA therapy.

Epidemiology: no data are available.

Clinical appearance: lesions are often multiple, asymptomatic, dyschromic, and with irregular borders. Melanosis, particularly when occurring on the genitalia, can clinically mimic mucosal melanoma, creating concern in both the patient and the physician.

Clinical course: little is known about the natural history or the risk of developing melanoma. Most of the lesions remain stable over decades, and evolution into genital melanoma is rare and occurs in the elderly.

Diagnosis: it is generally made on the basis of clinical findings. Sometimes, multiple biopsies may be necessary to avoid misdiagnosis and to confirm the benign nature of the condition by the lack of atypical features on histopathological examination.

Therapy: for small lesions, which can easily be removed, surgery is the best option. Large or multiple lesions should be monitored with videodermatoscopy before planning treatment, to evaluate clinical changes such as enlargement or discoloration.

Suggested Reading

Cervigón I, Palomo A, Torres LM (2007) Melanotic macules of the penis. Actas Dermosifiliogr 98:722-3
Laguna C, Pitarch G, Roche E, Fortea JM (2006) Atypical pigmented penile macules. Actas Dermosifiliogr 97:470-2
Romero-Maté A, Miñano-Medrano R, Nájera-Botello L et al (2010) Reticulate genital pigmentation associated with localized vitiligo. Arch Dermatol 146:574-5
Sopena Barona J, Gamo Villegas R, Guerra Tapia A, Iglesias Díez L (2003) Acromelanosis. An Pediatr 58:277-80

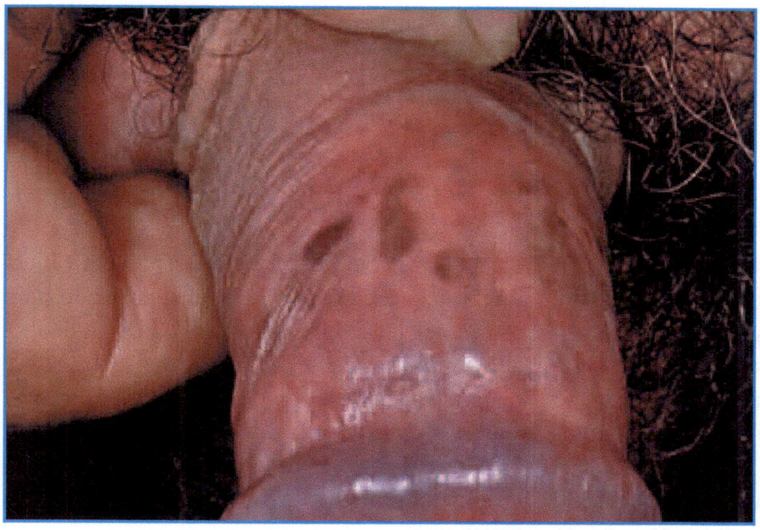

Fig. 6.5 Multiple, oval-shaped, and brownish macules on the inner foreskin

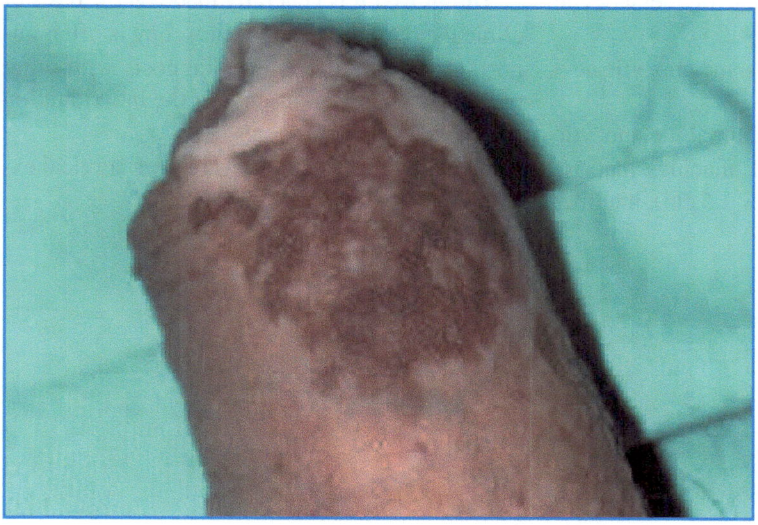

Fig. 6.6 Multiple and confluent brownish macules on the shaft

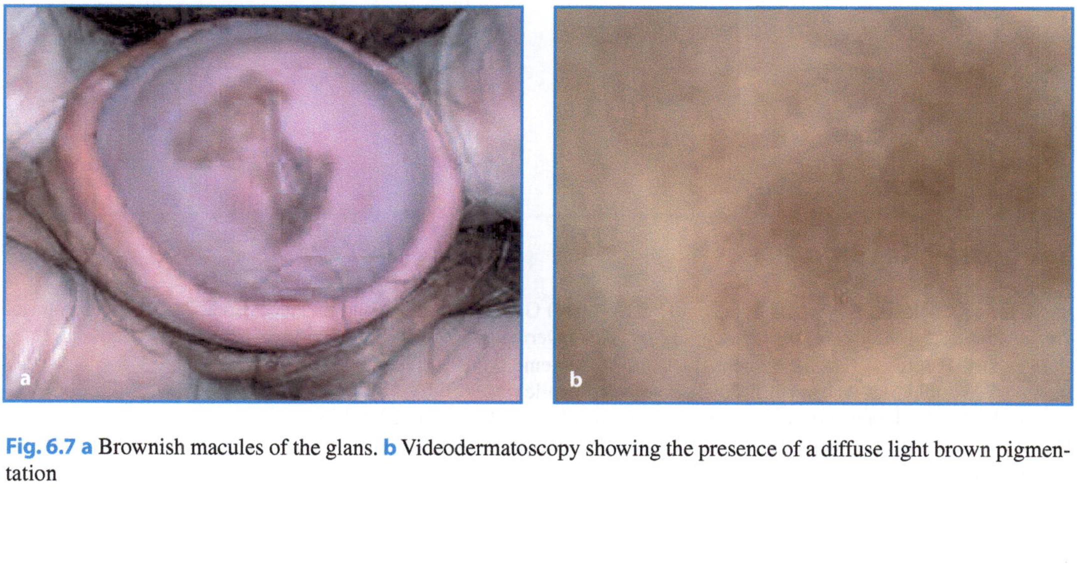

Fig. 6.7 a Brownish macules of the glans. **b** Videodermatoscopy showing the presence of a diffuse light brown pigmentation

Melanocytic Nevi

Definition: congenital and acquired melanocytic nevi are respectively benign neoplasms or hamartomas, composed of melanocytes. In acquired lesions, nevus cells may form some peculiar clusters at the dermal junction (junctional nevi), in the dermis (dermal and blue nevi), or in both (compound nevi).

Etiology: it remains unknown. Both genetic and environmental (sun exposure) factors seem to be involved in the development of melanocytic nevi.

Epidemiology: on the penis, melanocytic nevi are very common.

Clinical appearance: congenital melanocytic nevi appear as brown to dark macules that are commonly classified as small (< 1.5 cm), intermediate (1.5-20 cm), or large/giant (>20 cm). Junctional nevi are sharply marginated, tan to dark brown macules, only a few millimiters in diameter. Compound and dermal nevi are soft, sharply marginated, and brown to skin colored. Blue nevi are bluish to gray-brown papules.

Clinical course: it is general benign, but some lesions may be at risk of developing malignant melanoma.

Diagnosis: it is generally made on the basis of clinical examination. Dermatoscopy is often important for the differential diagnosis with other pigmented skin lesions and for the individuation of atypical lesions.

Therapy: atypical lesions require surgical excision.

Suggested Reading

El Shabrawi-Caelen L, Soyer HP, Schaeppi H et al (2004) Genital lentigines and melanocytic nevi with superimposed lichen sclerosus: a diagnostic challenge. J Am Acad Dermatol 50:690-4

Hengge UR, Meurer M (2005) Pigmented lesions of the genital mucosa. Hautarzt 56:540-9

Mahto M, Woolley PD, Ashworth J (2004) Pigmented penile macules. Int J STD AIDS 15:717-9

Schärer L (2007) Melanocytic nevi at special anatomical sites. Pathologie 28:430-6

Val-Bernal JF, Val D, Garijo MF (2009) Clinically unapparent melanocytic nevi on the prepuce. J Cutan Pathol 36:444-7

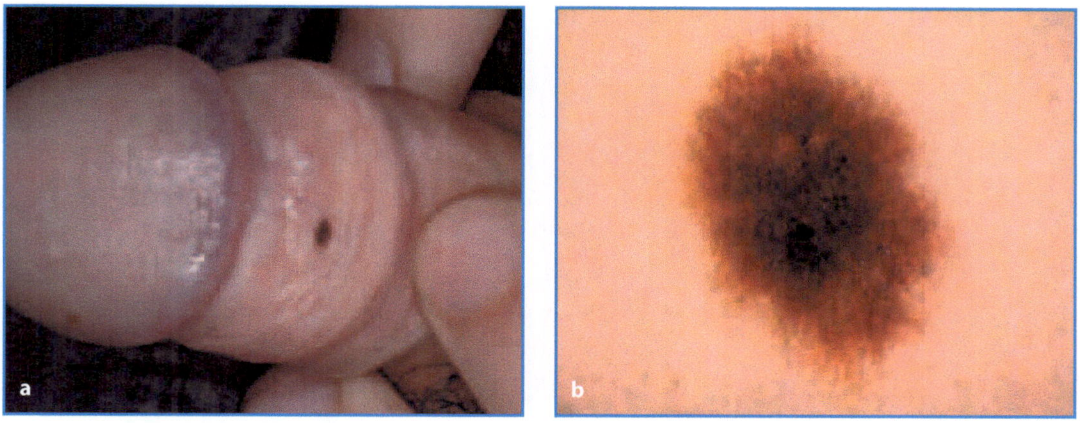

Fig. 6.8 Junctional melanocytic nevus. a Small, roundish, and hyperpigmented patch of the inner foreskin. b Videodermatoscopy showing the presence of a uniform dark pigmentation and multiple black dots

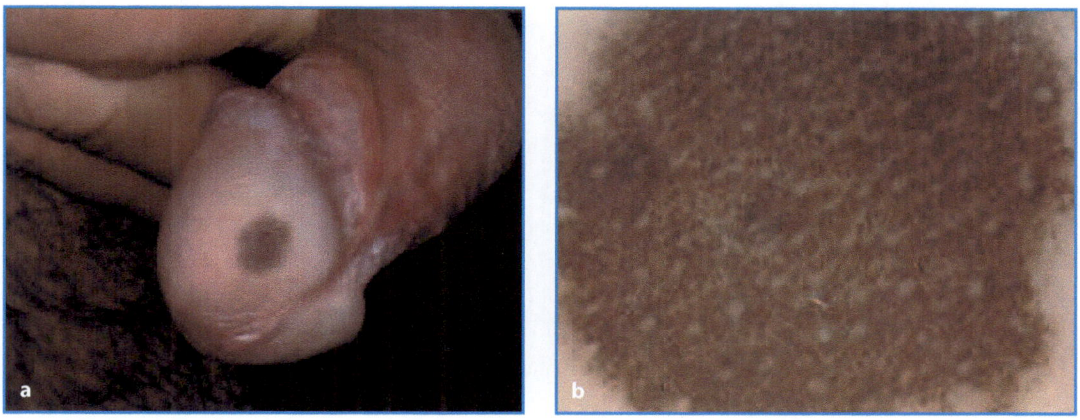

Fig. 6.9 Compound melanocytic nevus. a Roundish and brown plaque of the glans. b Videodermatoscopy showing the presence of a regular, diffuse, and globular pattern

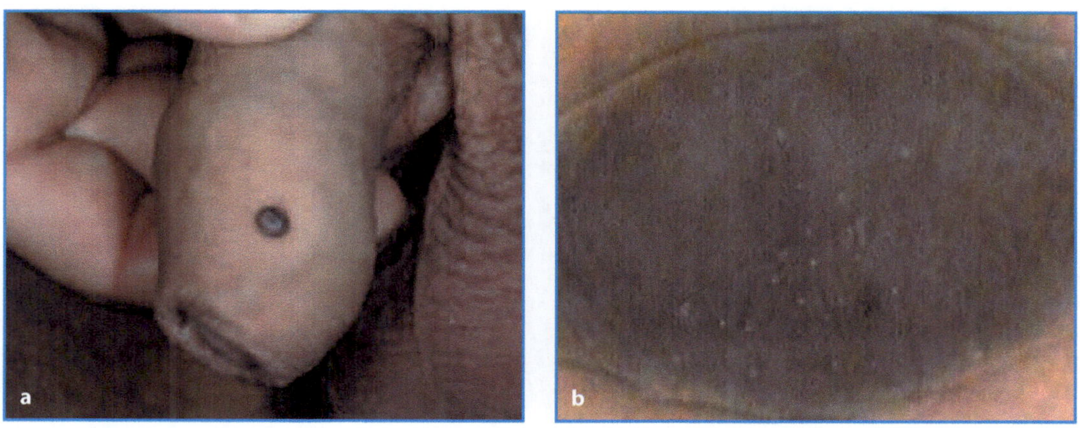

Fig. 6.10 Blue nevus. a Small and bluish papule of the shaft. b Videodermatoscopy showing the presence of homogeneous blue pigmentation

7 Benign Neoplastic Disorders

Pompeo Donofrio, Paola Donofrio, Piera Catalfo,
and Giuseppe Micali

P. Donofrio (✉)
School of Dermatology and Venereology
"Federico II" University of Naples, Naples, Italy
e-mail: dermodonofrio@hotmail.it

G. Micali et al., *Atlas of Male Genital Disorders*,
DOI: 10.1007/978-88-470-2787-9_7, © Springer-Verlag Italia 2013

Pearly Penile Papules

Definition: pearly penile papules, also known as hirsuties papillaris genitalis, are angiofibromatous lesions localized at the glans sulcus and corona. They are considered a normal anatomic variant.

Etiology: it is unknown.

Epidemiology: they do not show any racial predilection. The prevalence of pearly penile papules is not well known, but it occurs in 10% to 50% of men. They are more common in young and uncircumcised men, with a peak of incidence between 20 and 30 years of age.

Clinical appearance: they are small, filiform or digitate, asymptomatic skin-coloured lesions arranged in encircling rows on the glans sulcus and corona.

Clinical course: they are benign tumors that do not cause any problems.

Diagnosis: the clinical feature is enough for diagnosis. At dermatoscopy, pearly penile papules appear as regular whitish pink cobblestone- or grape-like structures in a few rows which may present central dotted or comma-like vessels in each papule.

Therapy: no treatment is needed.

Suggested Reading

Kluger N, Dereure O (2009) Images in clinical medicine. Penile papules. N Engl J Med 26;360:1336
Monroe JR (2009) Does this man have genital warts? Pearly penile papules. JAAPA 22:16
Ozeki M, Saito R, Tanaka M (2008) Dermoscopic features of pearly penile papules. Dermatology 217:21-2
Rokhsar CK, Ilyas H (2008) Fractional resurfacing for the treatment of pearly penile papules. Dermatol Surg 34:1420-2
Watanabe T, Yoshida Y, Yamamoto O (2010) Differential diagnosis of pearly penile papules and penile condyloma acuminatum by dermoscopy. Eur J Dermatol 20:414-5

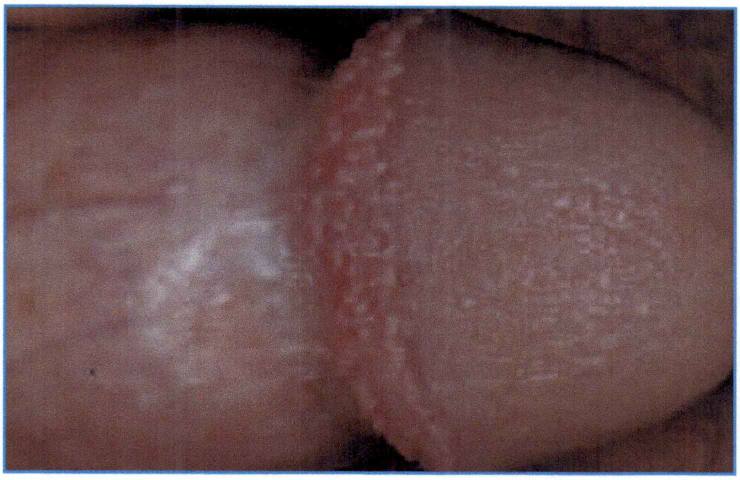

Fig. 7.1 Multiple, regular, small, and skin colored papules on the corona

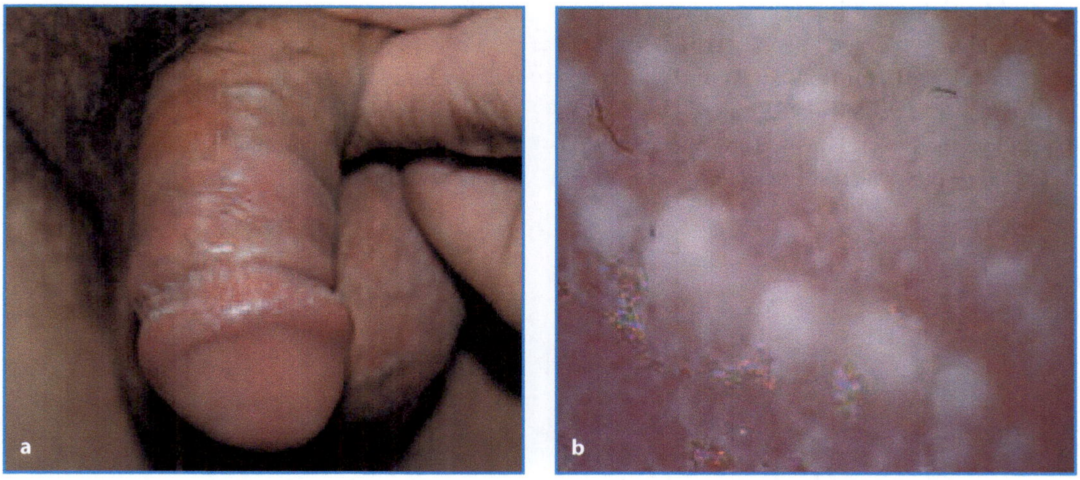

Fig. 7.2 a Small and whitish papules arranged in encircling rows on the corona. b Videodermatoscopy (X30) showing the presence of regular, whitish, and linearly arranged structures

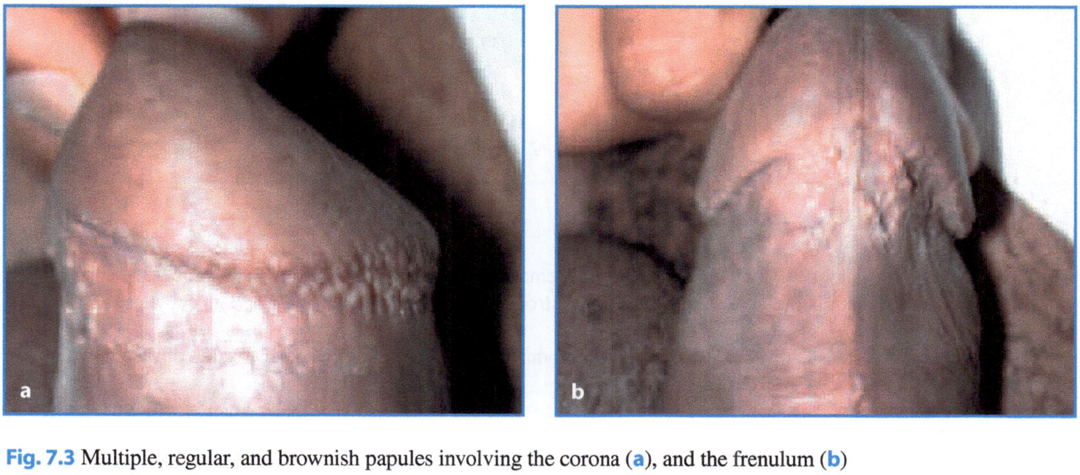

Fig. 7.3 Multiple, regular, and brownish papules involving the corona (a), and the frenulum (b)

Fibroepithelial Polyp

Definition: a fibroepithelial polyp, also known as a skin tag, is a cutaneous pedunculated lesion made of lax fibrous tissue, generally localized in the flexural surface of the skin, such as neck, axillae and inguinal folds.

Etiology: it is unknown, but the prevalence of fibroepithelial polyps increases with advancing age.

Epidemiology: it is a very common condition in middle- and old-aged people of both sexes.

Clinical appearance: they present with one or more cutaneous pedunculated lesions generally localized on the flexural areas. They appear as skin-coloured or pigmented soft lesions, with a smooth or papillomatous surface. They are asymptomatic, but they can become painful when inflamed.

Clinical course: the number and the size of the lesions increase with advancing age, but in any case remain benign. After torsion around the peduncle, the lesions can become bigger, darker, painful, and necrotizing.

Diagnosis: the clinical appearance is enough for diagnosis.

Therapy: as these are benign lesions, a specific therapy is not needed, but they can be removed for aesthetic and/or functional reasons. Surgical ablation, cryotherapy, cauterization, and laser therapy can be useful.

Suggested Reading

Fetsch JF, Davis CJ Jr, Hallman JR et al (2004) Lymphedematous fibroepithelial polyps of the glans penis and prepuce: a clinicopathologic study of 7 cases demonstrating a strong association with chronic condom catheter use. Hum Pathol 35:190-5

Rodríguez Collar TL, Valdés Estévez B, López Marín L, Soranyer Horroutinel Scull R (2010) Penile fibroepithelial polyp. Case report. Arch Esp Urol 63:309-12

Tsai TF, Hung CS, Hsiao CH (2008) Fibroepithelial polyp of glans penis in a man who practiced genital hanging kung fu. J Am Acad Dermatol 59:S35-7

Turgut M, Yenilmez A, Can C et al (2005) Fibroepithelial polyp of glans penis. Urology 65:593

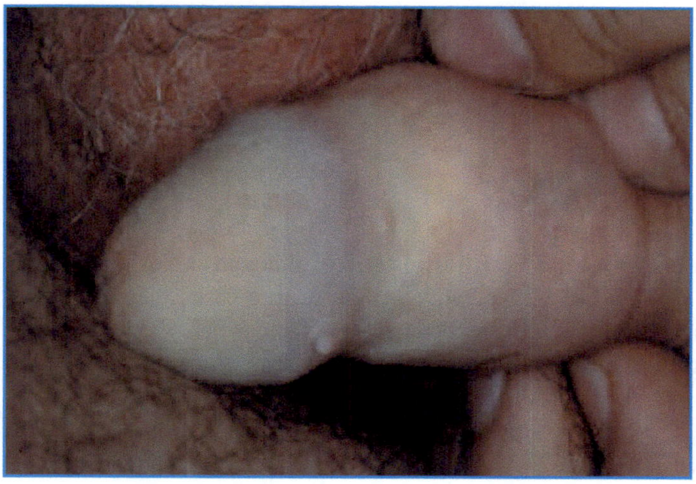

Fig. 7.4 Skin-colored, soft, fleshy, and pedunculated lesion arising from the corona

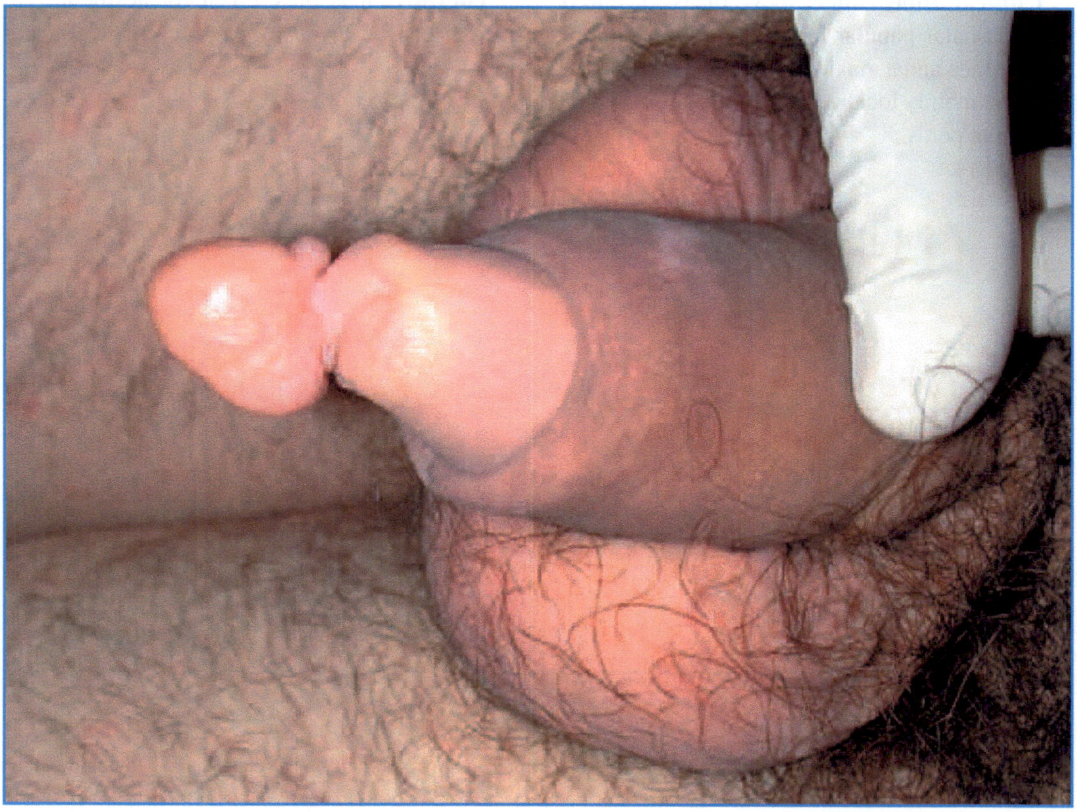

Fig. 7.5 Giant lesion arising from the foreskin

Angiokeratoma

Definition: angiokeratoma is a vascular expansion with a hyperkeratotic surface.

Etiology: it is the result of the dilatation of dermal papillae vessels. Possible pathogenetic mechanisms include venous hypertension, vascular malformations and vascular fragility.

Epidemiology: genital angiokeratomas are very frequent in adult patients, appearing at about 30-40 years of age.

Clinical appearance: they consist of one or more vascular papular lesions with a hyperkeratotic surface and a maximum diameter of 1-5 mm. They are mainly localized on the scrotum, less often on the penis.

Clinical course: although angiokeratomas are generally benign, in rare cases they can reveal systemic disorders, such as Fabry's disease.

Diagnosis: it is generally clinical. At dermatoscopy, angiokeratoma is characterized by the presence of a whitish veil and red or dark lacunae. A histopathological examination can be helpful in certain cases to distinguish angiokeratomas from other vascular tumors.

Therapy: it is only given for aesthetic reasons. It can be given by electric coagulation or laser.

Suggested Reading

Feramisco JD, Fournier JB, Zedek DC, Venna SS (2009) Eruptive angiokeratomas on the glans penis. Dermatol Online J 15:14

Leis-Dosil VM, Alijo-Serrano F, Aviles-Izquierdo JA et al (2007) Angiokeratoma of the glans penis: clinical, histopathological and dermoscopic correlation. Dermatol Online J 1:13-19

Micali G, Lacarrubba F (2011) Augmented diagnostic capability using videodermatoscopy on selected infectious and non-infectious penile growths. Int J Dermatol 50:1501-5

Pavone P, Lucenti C, Fraggetta F et al (2008) Congenital lymphedema-lymphangiectasia associated with scrotal angiokeratoma (Fordyce Type) and hearing impairment. J Clin Gastroenterol 42:715-9

Rees R, Freeman A, Malone P et al (2009) Case study: the surgical management of angiokeratoma resulting from radiotherapy for penile cancer. ScientificWorldJournal 9:339-42

Saha M, Barlow R, Bunker CB (2006) Angiokeratoma circumscriptum of the penis. Br J Dermatol 154:775-6

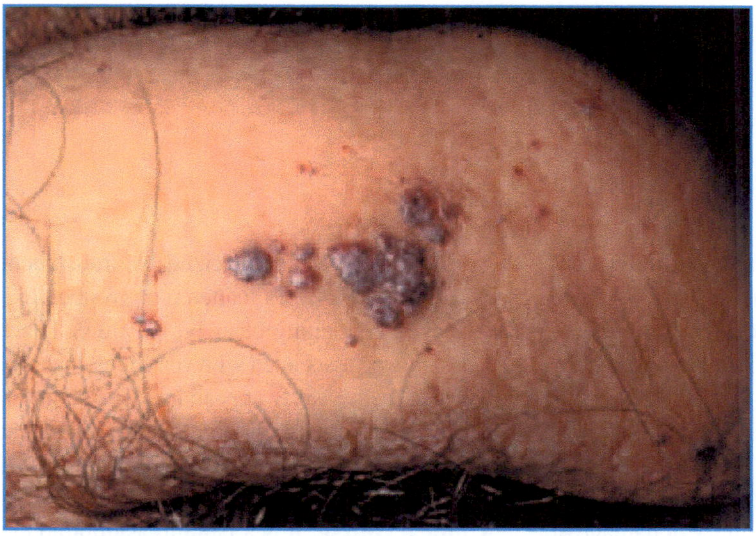

Fig. 7.6 Dark reddish papules on the shaft

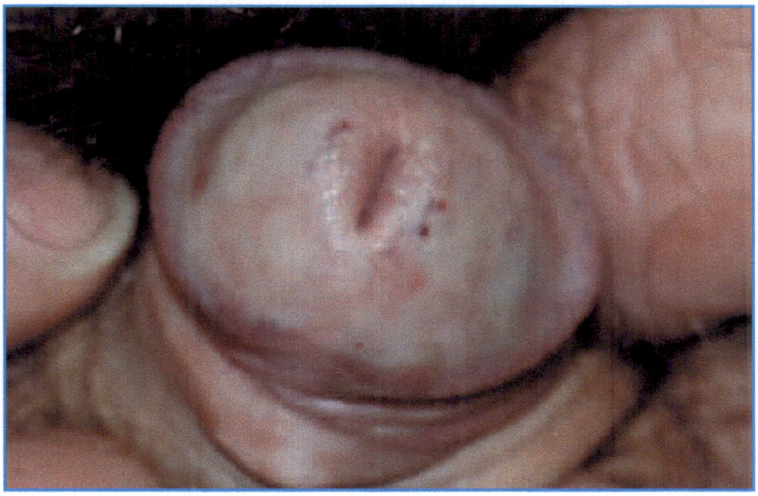

Fig. 7.7 Dark reddish papules on the glans

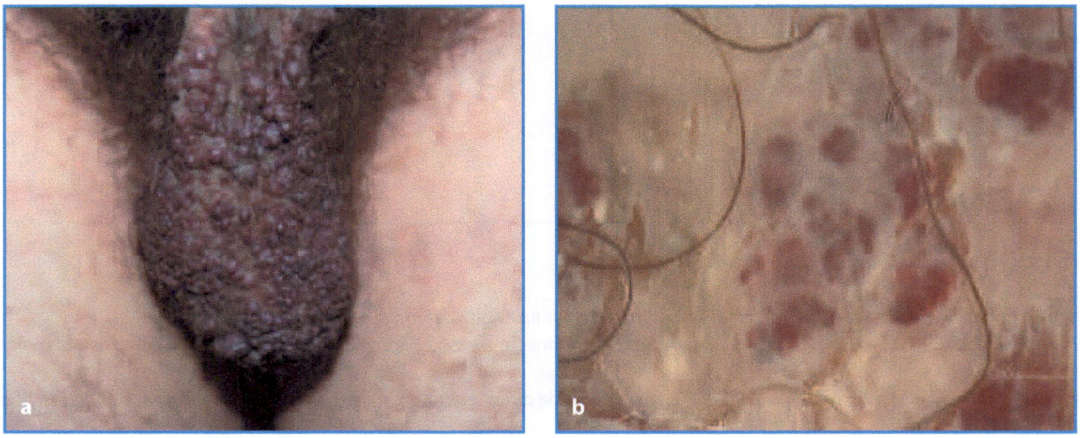

Fig. 7.8 **a** Several bluish papules on the scrotum and proximal shaft. **b** Videodermatoscopy showing the presence of red lacunae and a whitish veil

Lymphangiomas

Definition: lymphangiomas are uncommon, congenital, lymphatic hamartomas of the skin and subcutaneous tissues. When occurring on superficial vessels, they are called lymphangioma circumscriptum.

Etiology: they represent a collection of lymphatic lacunae separated from the normal network of lymphatic vessels. The forms that develop in adulthood are probably due to injury or damage of the deep collecting channels, leading to lymph stasis with backflow resulting in subsequent dilation of the upper dermal lymphatics.

Epidemiology: they account for about 5% of all vascular tumors and 25% of all benign vascular tumors in children. They are more common in females than in males.

Clinical appearance: lymphangioma circumscriptum, which may arise at birth, in childhood or in adolescence, is characterized by translucent vesicles of varying sizes scattered or grouped like frog spawn, containing clear lymph fluid. These vesicles may be associated with verrucous changes, which give them a warty appearance. The common sites are axillary folds, shoulders, neck, proximal part of the limbs, and oral cavity. Involvement of the scrotum and penis may also be observed.

Clinical course: it is a benign, asymptomatic and often negligible condition.

Diagnosis: the clinical feature is generally evocative for diagnosis. Ultrasonography may be helpful in patients who have suspicious deep extension of the lesions.

Therapy: no treatment is needed. Patients usually seek medical treatment for cosmetic reasons. Incomplete excision can result in recurrence.

Suggested Reading

Grossgold ET, Kusuda L (2007) Scrotal lymphangioma in an adult. Urology 70:590

Lee WC, Park SB, Lee JH et al (2009) Sonographic findings in a case of scrotal lymphangioma in a 68-year-old male. J Clin Ultrasound 37:428-30

Pal DK, Banerjee M, Moulik D et al (2010) Lymphangioma circumscriptum of the scrotum following vasectomy. Indian J Urol 26:294-5

Rastogi R, Meena GL, Kumar R, Rastogi V (2010) Cystic lymphangioma scroti: a common tumor at a rare location. Saudi J Kidney Dis Transpl 21:1132-4

Wong R, Melnyk M, Tang SS, Nguan C (2012) Scrotal lymphangiomatosis: a case report. Can Urol Assoc J 6:E11-4

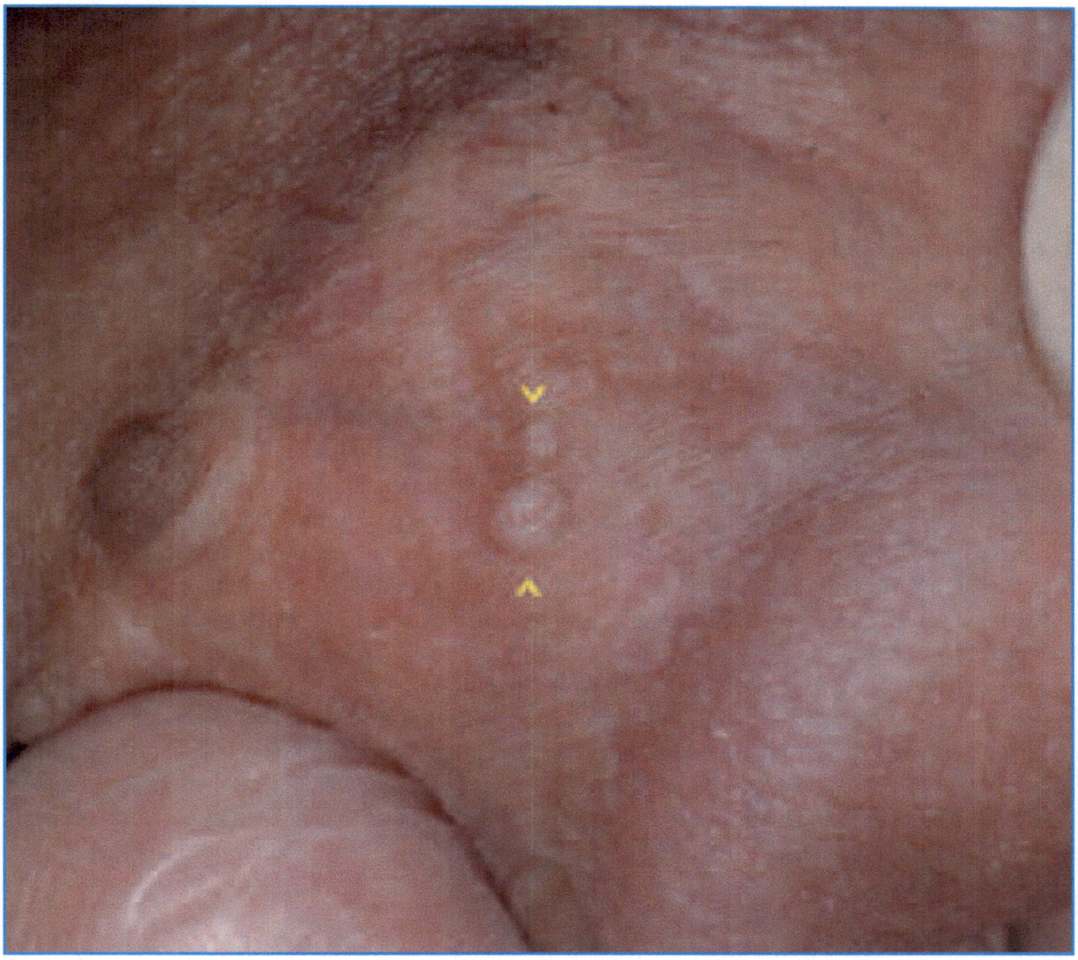

Fig. 7.9 Lymphangioma circumscriptum: small and translucent vesicles on the coronal sulcus

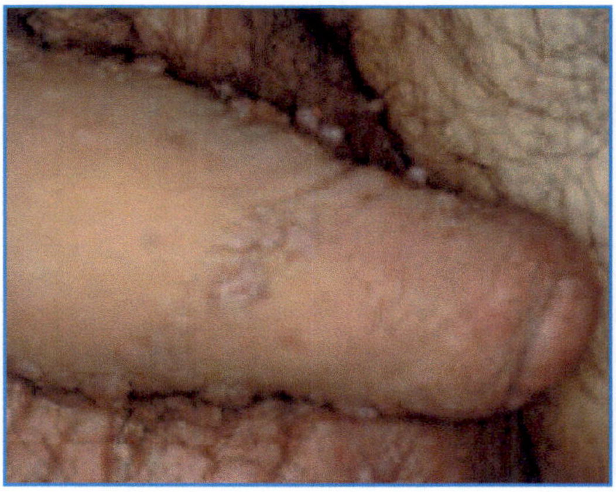

Fig. 7.10 Lymphangioma circumscriptum: multiple and warty vesicles on the penis and the scrotum

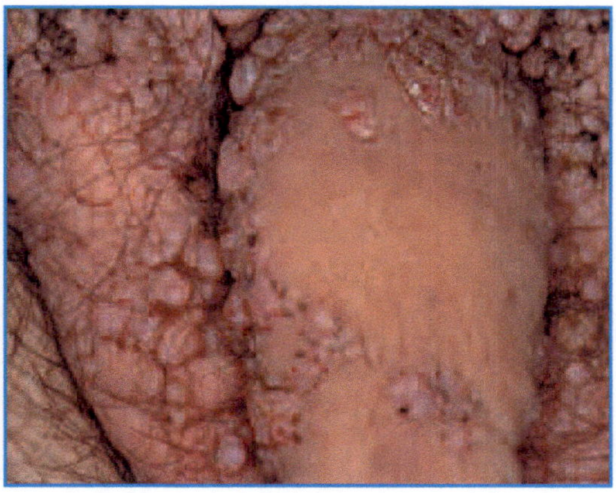

Fig. 7.11 Lymphangioma circumscriptum: multiple and confluent warty vesicles on the penis and the scrotum

Seborrheic Keratosis

Definition: seborrheic keratosis, also known as seborrheic wart, is a benign epithelial skin tumor.

Etiology: it is unclear, but older age and sun exposure are considered exogenous risk factors. The possibility of a genetic predisposition has been suggested.

Epidemiology: it is one of the most frequent skin tumours, but detailed epidemiological data are lacking. It is more common among Caucasians, with no gender predilection. Its prevalence increases with advancing age.

Clinical appearance: it is a well-demarcated, roundish or oval raised papule, with verrucous, uneven, or dull surface. At its onset, it can be flat with a smooth, velvety surface, growing thicker over time. The colour varies from yellowish to gray-brown or black. The lesion can be single, but multiple elements of sizes ranging from a few millimetres to several centimetres are often found. Seborrheic keratosis can appear anywhere in the body, except the palmoplantar areas.

Clinical course: with advancing age, the number and size of the lesions increase. After removal they can relapse, but do not show any malignant potential.

Diagnosis: it is usually straightforward, based on the clinical appearance. Dermatoscopy shows the presence of milia-like cysts and comedo-like openings on a background varying from opaque light-brown to dark-brown or black. Histopathological examination may sometimes be necessary to rule out melanocytic tumors or bowenoid papulosis.

Therapy: as this is a benign condition, specific treatment is not necessary, but seborrheic keratosis can be removed for aesthetic and functional reasons. They can be treated by curettage, shaving, cryotherapy, electric cautery or laser therapy.

Suggested Reading

De Roos KP, Bruins FG (2008) Giant genital seborrheic keratosis or Buschke Löwenstein tumor? Dermatol Surg 34:15-16

Livaoglu M, Karacal N, Gücer H, Arvas L (2007) Giant genital seborrheic keratosis. Dermatol Surg 33:1357-8

Tardío JC, Bancalari E, Moreno A, Martín-Fragueiro LM (2012) Genital seborrheic keratoses are human papillomavirus-related lesions. A linear array genotyping test study. APMIS 120:477-83

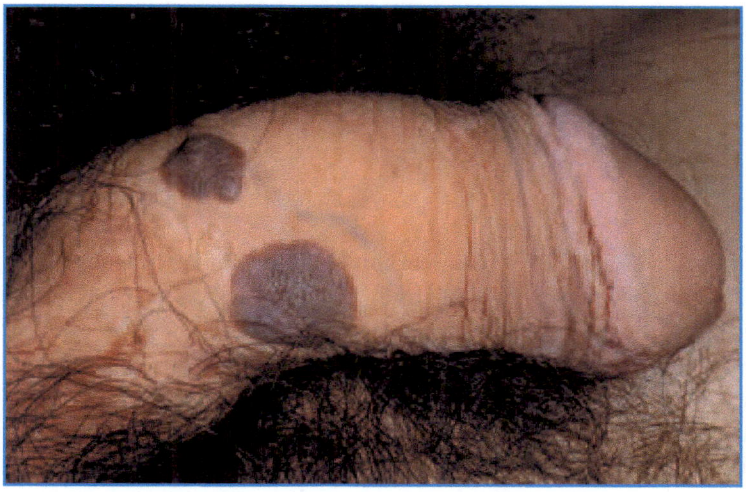

Fig. 7.12 Brown, roundish, well-demarcated, and verrucous lesions on the shaft

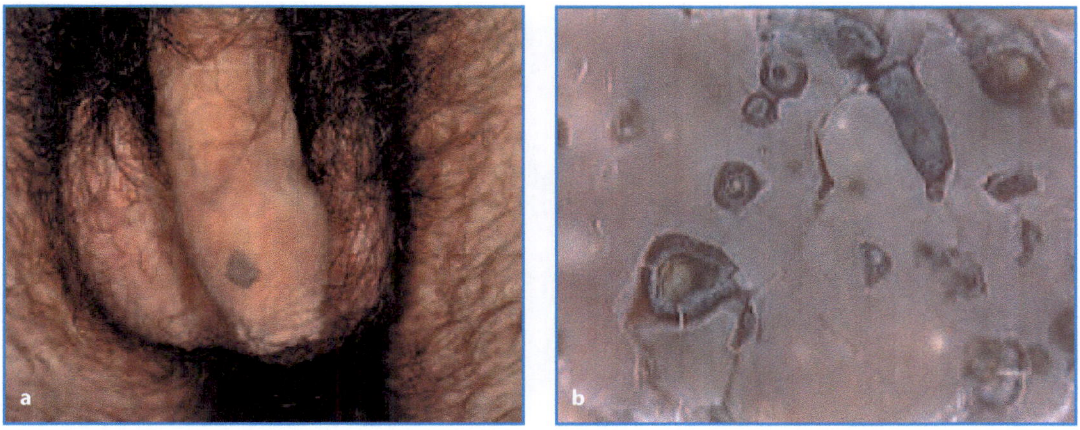

Fig. 7.13 a Brown, roundish, and verrucous lesion on the penis. **b** Videodermatoscopy (X30) showing the presence of milia-like cysts and comedo-like openings on a light-brown background

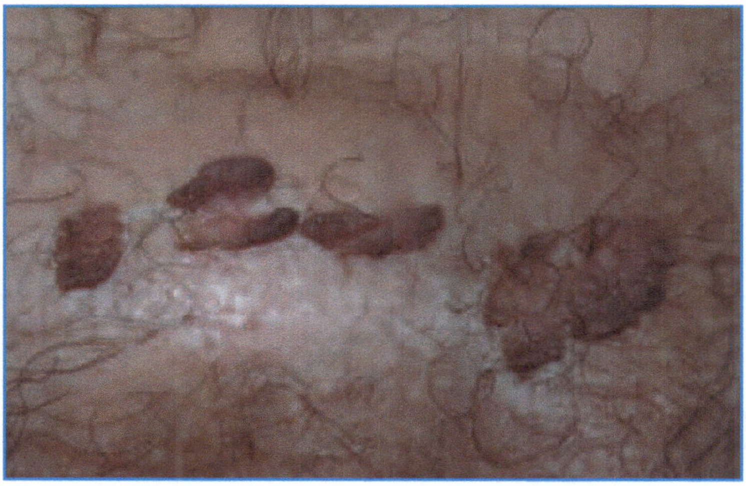

Fig. 7.14 Light brown, smooth, and papillomatous lesions on the groin

Penile Horn

Definition: the term penile horn indicates a protruding hyperkeratotic penile lesion, conical in shape with an erythematous base.

Etiology: it is not well known, but chronic irritation, radiation, and traumas are implicated. The most important etiological factor is considered to be long-lasting phimosis with chronic preputial inflammation.

Epidemiology: it is a rare condition, with approximately 140 cases reported in the literature.

Clinical appearance: it generally presents as a keratotic, yellowish, roundish, raised lesion with an erythematous base.

Clinical course: the condition is benign in 40-60% of cases, but some authors consider penile horns as premalignant lesions.

Diagnosis: differential diagnosis includes squamous cell carcinoma, genital warts, keratoacanthoma, or benign hyperplastic epithelium, which may present as a penile horn. Histopathological examination is mandatory.

Therapy: various physical treatments, such as electric coagulative ablation, cryotherapy, and ablative laser therapy may be used. Considering the possibility of a malignant lesion, surgical excision with histopathological examination is indicated.

Suggested Reading

Nayyar R, Singh P, Seth A (2009) Penile cutaneous horn over long standing radiation dermatitis. J Postgrad Med 55:287
Ponce de León J, Algaba F, Salvador J (1994) Cutaneous horn of glans penis. Br J Urol 74:257-8
Vera-Donoso CD, Lujan S, Gomez L et al (2009) Cutaneous horn in glans penis: a new clinical case. Scand J Urol Nephrol 43:92-3

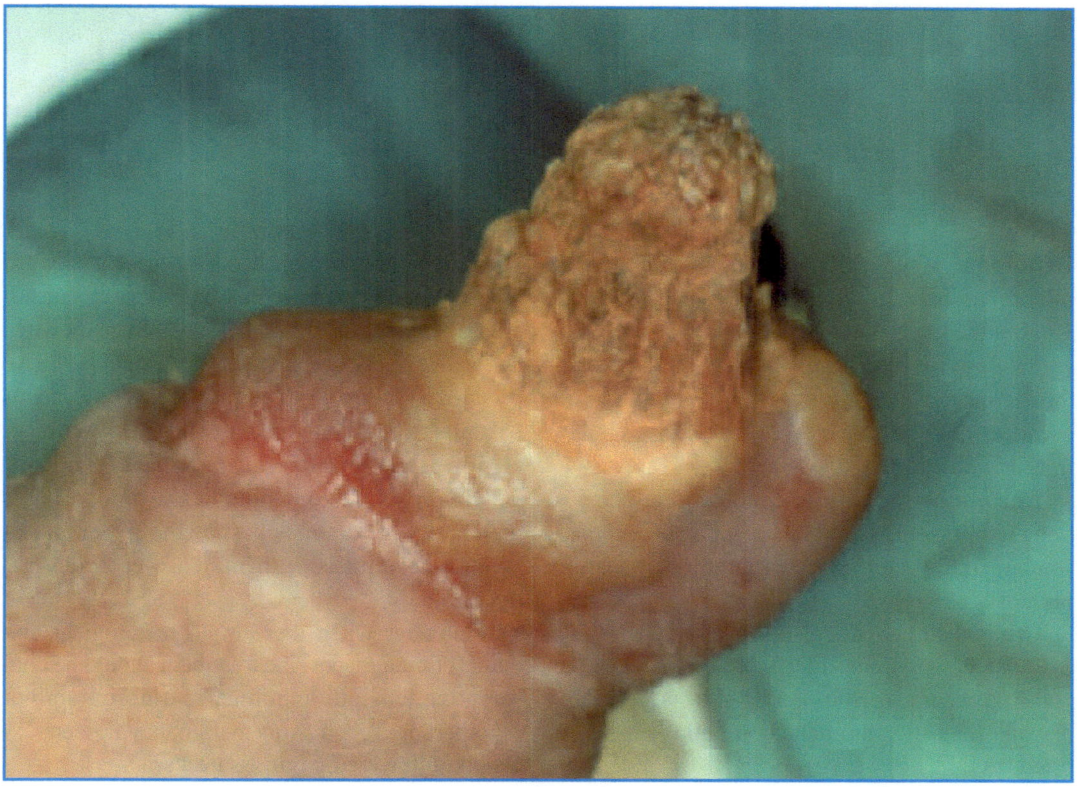

Fig. 7.15 Keratotic, yellowish, and raised lesion developing from the glans

Pseudoepitheliomatous Keratotic and Micaceous Balanitis

Definition: pseudoepitheliomatous keratotic and micaceous balanitis is a rare penile disease involving the glans in advanced age.

Etiology: it is not well known, but some authors consider it as a form of pyodermatitis or a pseudoepitheliomatous response to various infections.

Epidemiology: it is an extremely rare condition affecting elderly men who undergo circumcison late in life, for the treatment of a pre-existing phimosis.

Clinical appearance: thick keratotic lesions associated with mica-like scales involving the glans are characteristic. Penile skin is generally dry and inelastic, and balanopreputial adhesions often occur.

Clinical course: the lesions have a prolonged course of many years. This was originally considered a benign dermatosis, but it was later shown to be capable of invasive growth. Some authors believe pseudoepitheliomatous keratotic and micaceous balanitis to be an intermediate stage between a benign hyperplasia and a squamous cell carcinoma.

Diagnosis: histopathological examination is mandatory for diagnosis, showing hyperkeratosis and acanthosis with mild lower epidermal dysplasia.

Therapy: when there is no histological evidence of malignancy, the treatment should be conservative, including topical 5-fluorouracil or cryotherapy. When overt malignancy is seen, excision with wide margins is necessary.

Suggested Reading

Bashir SJ, Grant JW, Burrows NP (2010) Pseudoepitheliomatous, keratotic and micaceous balanitis after penile squamous cell carcinoma. Clin Exp Dermatol 35:749-51

Pai VV, Hanumanthayya K, Naveen KN et al (2010) Pseudoepitheliomatous, keratotic, and micaceous balanitis presenting as cutaneous horn in an adult male. Indian J Dermatol Venereol Leprol 76:547-9

Perry D, Lynch PJ, Fazel N (2008) Pseudoepitheliomatous, keratotic, and micaceous balanitis: case report and review of the literature. Dermatol Nurs 20:117-20

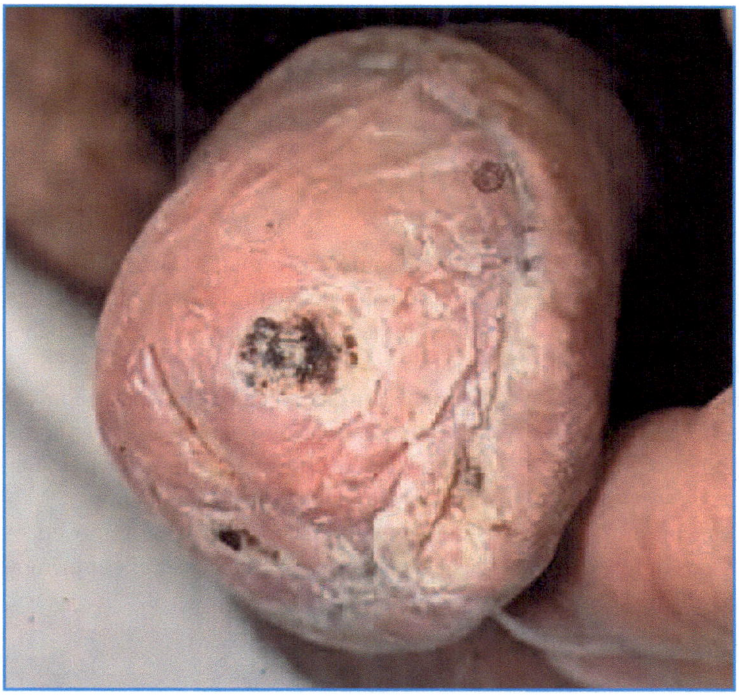

Fig. 7.16 Thick keratotic lesions associated with mica-like scales involving the glans and the foreskin

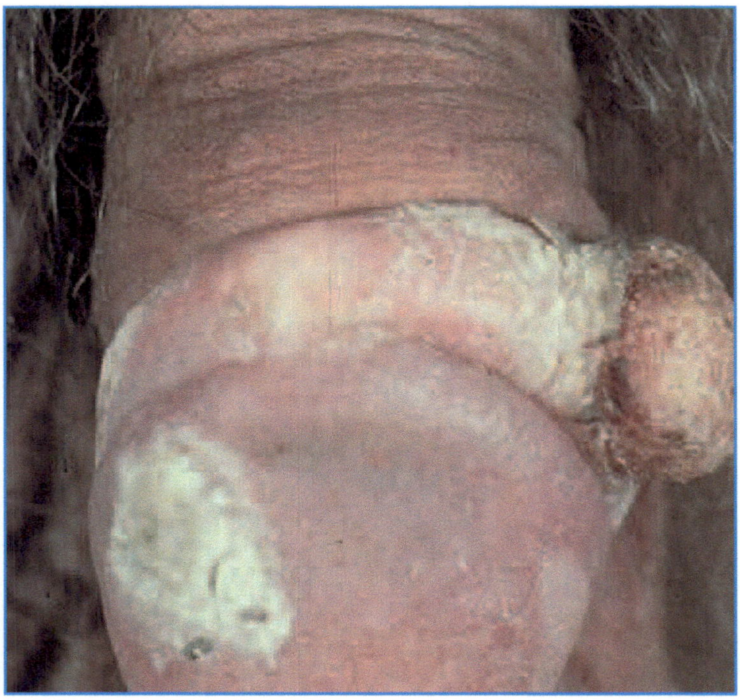

Fig. 7.17 Evolution towards invasive squamous cell carcinoma of the foreskin

Leukoplakia

Definition: leukoplakia is a precancerous condition of the visible mucous membranes.

Etiology: in oral leukoplakia a pathogenetic role is probably played by chronic irritation from cigarette smoke, ill-fitting dentures, or dental angles, and in genital leukoplakia from oncogenic HPV infection, poor genital hygiene, and lack of circumcision.

Epidemiology: it is often seen on oral mucosa, and rarely observed on the glans or foreskin. It mostly affects middle-aged and elderly men.

Clinical appearance: it presents as an asymptomatic whitish patch with clear-cut edges. It must be differentiated from lichen planus and lichen sclerosus.

Clinical course: if untreated, the lesion can evolve into an invasive squamous cell carcinoma.

Diagnosis: the clinical diagnosis must be confirmed by histopathological examination.

Therapy: the lesion should be removed by surgical excision, electric cautery, or laser therapy.

Suggested Reading

Kolde G, Vakilzadeh F (1983) Leukoplakia of the prepuce with epidermolytic hyperkeratosis: a case report. Acta Derm Venereol 63:571-3

Mikhail GR (1980) Cancers, precancers, and pseudocancers on the male genitalia. A review of clinical appearances, histopathology, and management. J Dermatol Surg Oncol 6:1027-35

Sakoda R, Oka M, Nakashima K (1978) Leukoplakia of the penis-bleomycin treatment. Br J Urol 50:355

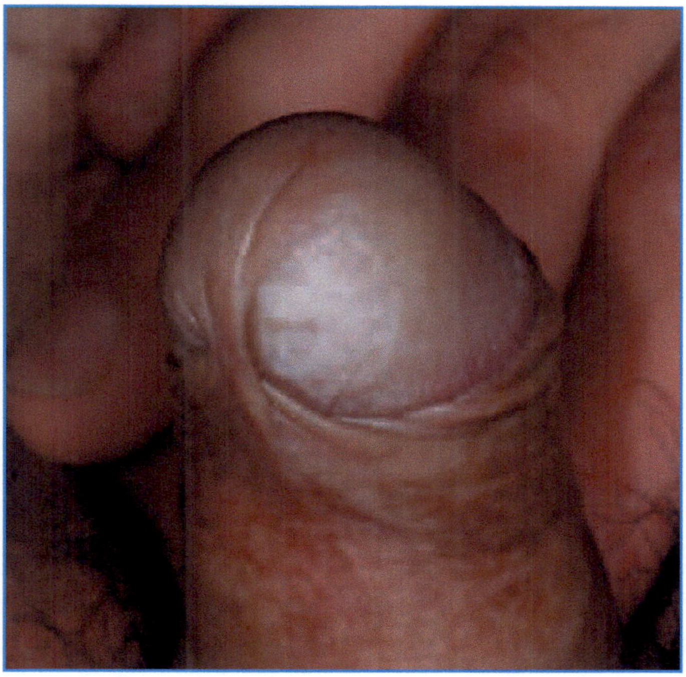

Fig. 7.18 Whitish and well-demarcated plaque on the glans

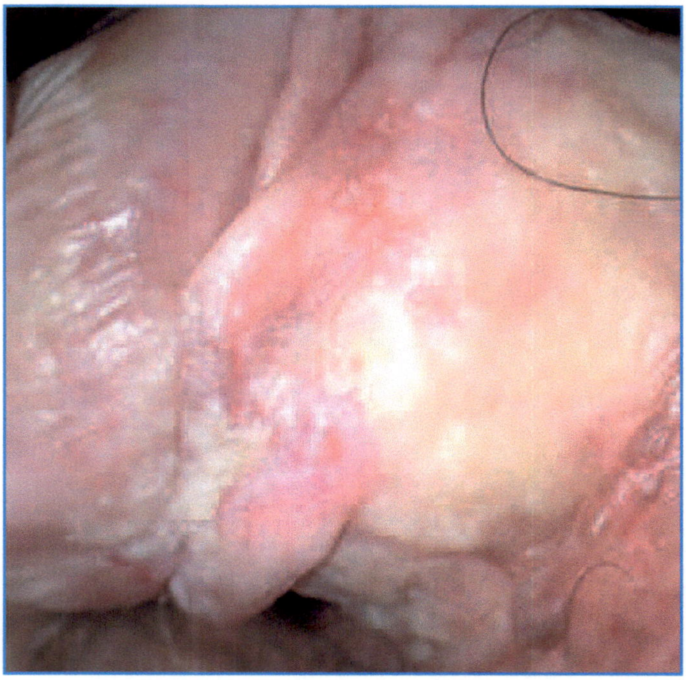

Fig. 7.19 White, roundish, and slightly raised lesion on the foreskin

8 Malignant Neoplastic Disorders

Giuseppe Micali, Francesco Lacarrubba, Philip J. Cohen, and Robert A. Schwartz

G. Micali (✉)
Dermatology Unit
Dipartimento di Specialità Medico-Chirurgiche
AOU "Policlinico – Vittorio Emanuele"
Presidio "G. Rodolico", Catania, Italy
e-mail: gimicali1@hotmail.it

G. Micali et al. (eds.), *Atlas of Male Genital Disorders*,
DOI: 10.1007/978-88-470-2787-9_8, © Springer-Verlag Italia 2013

Kaposi's Sarcoma

Definition: Kaposi's Sarcoma (KS) is a proliferative process of vascular cells that are presumed to be endothelial in origin.

Etiology: it is caused by the newly discovered herpes type 8 (KSHV or HHV-8), a virus that may be transmitted sexually and by saliva.

Epidemiology: men are affected much more often than women. This is the most common neoplasm in those with acquired immunodeficiency syndrome (AIDS). It tends to appear on acral regions such as the lower legs; approximately 18% of AIDS patients with Kaposi's sarcoma will have lesions on the penis or genitalia.

Clinical appearance: KS occurs in several subtypes: a classical form in elderly men of Mediterranean origin; endemic disease in indigenous Africans; and as a rapidly disseminated disease in immunosuppressed individuals (HIV and transplanted patients). KS often involves the genitalia as part of a disseminated cutaneous disease. In rare cases this neoplasm presents initially on the penis; a violaceous indurated lesion most often occurs on the glans. The cutaneous lesions of KS are multiform: red, brown, skin-colored, or violaceous patches, papules or plaques, frequently with linear borders. Ulceration may be present. Lesions occurring on the genitalia are often similar in appearance to those occurring elsewhere. KS on the skin often reflects systemic involvement, especially in the lymph nodes and intestine.

Clinical course: KS is usually asymptomatic, but it may cause emotional distress to the patient, especially if evident on the penis. Rarely, it may enlarge and infiltrate periurethral tissues, causing interference with urinary flow. Paradoxically, KS may worsen or first become apparent in association with the institution of antiretroviral therapy.

Diagnosis: the clinical picture of KS is often typical. Histological examination reveals a vascular tumor with proliferation of erythrocyte-filled vascular slits and blood vessels with prominent endothelial cells.

Therapy: it depends on the type and the degree of dissemination. Conservative therapy is recommended, with palliative radiotherapy or Nd:YAG laser treatment offering satisfactory local management. Individual cutaneous nodules can be treated with cryotherapy or intralesional injections of vinblastine. When possible, factors leading to the presence of immune suppression should be modified. Systemic chemotherapy or radiotherapy may be required if systemic disease is present.

Suggested Reading

D'Antuono A, Zauli S, Bellavista S et al (2012) AIDS-related Kaposi's sarcoma involving the genital and inguinal regions. Int J Dermatol [Epub ahead of print]

Micali G, Nasca MR, De Pasquale R, Innocenzi D (2003) Primary classic Kaposi's sarcoma of the penis: report of a case and review. J Eur Acad Dermatol Venereol 17:320-3

Schwartz RA, Cohen JB, Watson RA et al (2000) Penile Kaposi's sarcoma preceded by chronic penile lymphoedema. Br J Dermatol 142:153-6

Schwartz RA, Micali G, Nasca MR, Scuderi L (2008) Kaposi's sarcoma: a continuing conundrum. J Am Acad Dermatol 59:179-206

Zargari O (2006) Exclusive penile Kaposi's sarcoma: report of an HIV-negative man successfully treated with radiotherapy. J Eur Acad Dermatol Venereol 20:318-20

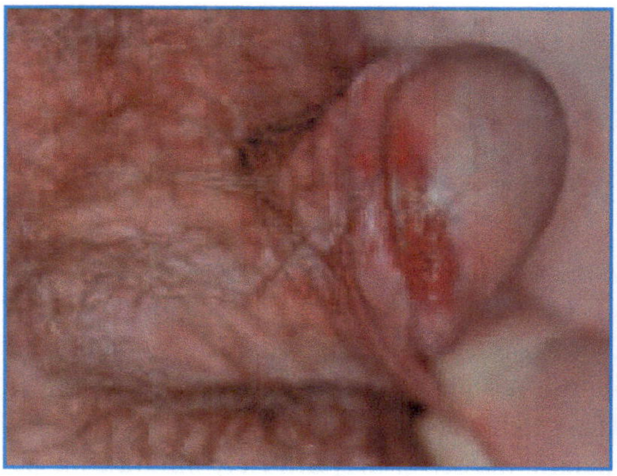

Fig. 8.1 Purplish patches and papules occurring on the corona

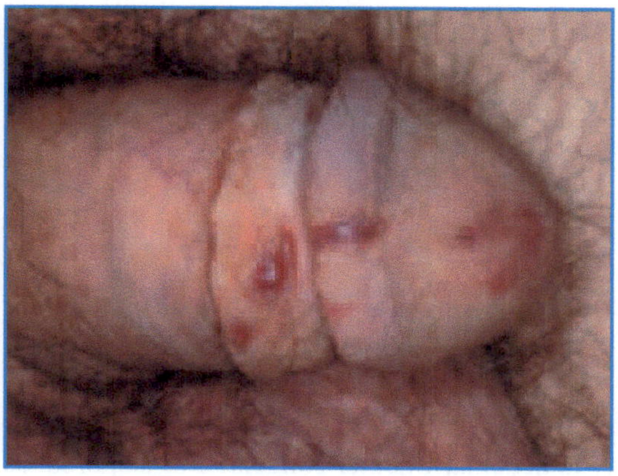

Fig. 8.2 Purplish patches involving the glans, the corona, and the foreskin

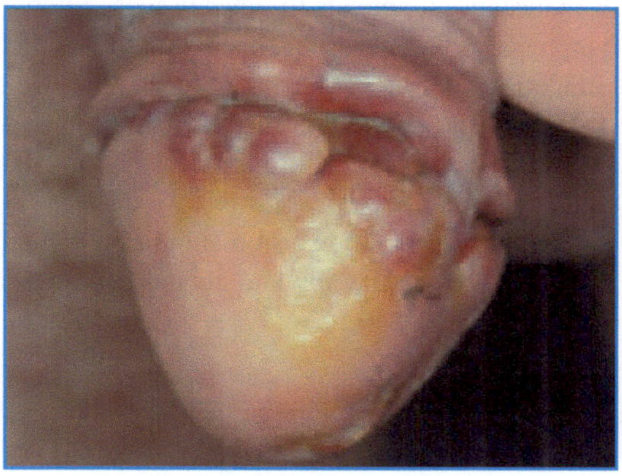

Fig. 8.3 Purplish nodules, linearly arranged on the corona, in an HIV+ patient

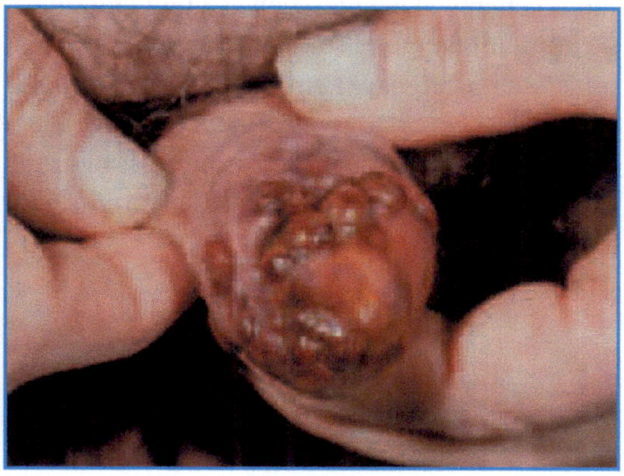

Fig. 8.4 Multicolored, confluent papules, and nodules on the glans

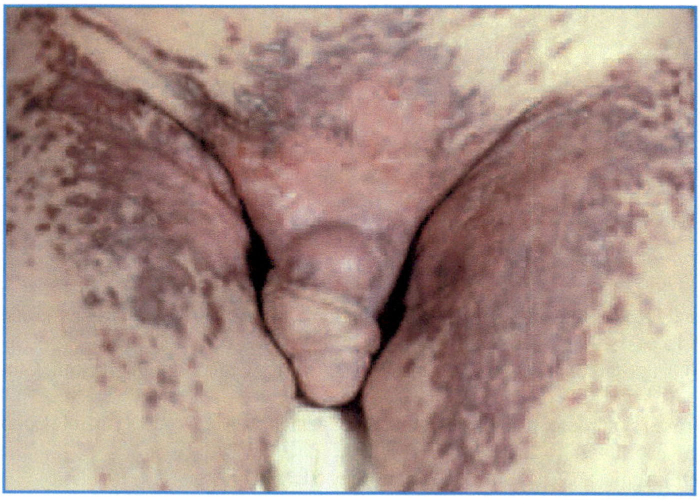

Fig. 8.5 Multiple lesions involving the genital area

Angiosarcoma

Definition: angiosarcoma is a malignant tumor of the vascular endothelium; it can have either cutaneous or visceral localization. It is often called the Stewart-Treves syndrome when it follows chronic lymphedema, whether congenital or acquired, as seen with some forms of filariasis.

Etiology: the most important causative agent is chronic lymphatic stasis; other possible predisposing factors are ionizing radiation and exposure to chemical agents, such as vinyl chloride.

Epidemiology: it is rare. It represents 1% of all soft tissue sarcomas. Females are more affected than males, especially when the angiosarcoma is preceded by lymphedema. Sporadic cases of penile angiosarcoma arising in the corpora cavernosa have been reported.

Clinical appearance: it is characterized by one or more hemorrhagic or vascular nodules and bluish-red plaques with ulcerative involvement. This tumor can form discrete painful or non-painful masses or may diffusely infiltrate the penis and adjacent structures. In contrast to angiosarcomas found elsewhere in the body, the majority of penile lesions tend to be indolent.

Clinical course: it may be primarily cutaneous or metastatic. It spreads to other tissues, notably lymph nodes, liver and lung, mainly through blood circulation.

Diagnosis: histopathological examination showing an atypical proliferation of endothelial cells is mandatory for diagnosis.

Therapy: surgical excision should be radical and prompt; radiotherapy and chemotherapy are less effective.

Suggested Reading

Calonje E, Fletcher CD, Wilson-Jones E et al (1994) Retiform hemangioendothelioma. A distinctive form of low-grade angiosarcoma delineated in a series of 15 cases. Am J Surg Pathol 18:115-25

Chiu LS, Wong KH, Lam WY et al (2006) Angiosarcoma of the scrotum after treatment of cancer of the rectum. Clin Exp Dermatol 31:706-7

Sharma A, Schwartz RA (2012) Stewart-Treves syndrome: pathogenesis and management. J Am Acad Dermatol [Epub ahead of print]

Webber RJ, Alsaffar N, Bissett D et al (1998) Angiosarcoma of the penis. Urology 51:130-1

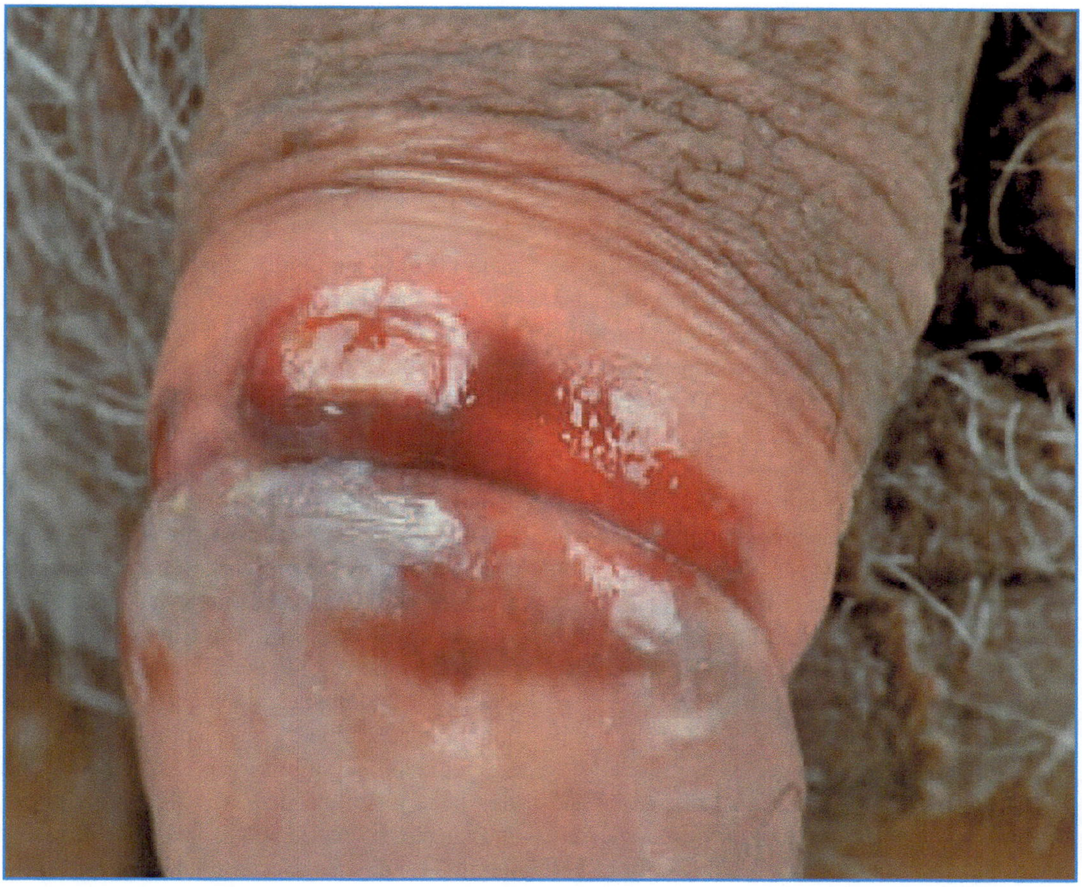

Fig. 8.6 Dark red, irregular, and hemorrhagic patch involving the glans and the inner foreskin

In Situ Carcinomas

Extramammary Paget's Disease

Definition: Extramammary Paget's Disease (EMPD) is a slow-growing epithelial neoplasm that occurs predominantly in apocrine gland-bearing skin. It is a rare intraepidermal apocrine carcinoma.

Etiology: it is unknown. The tumor probably arises from pluripotent germinative cells in the apocrine sweat glands that are able to differentiate into many kinds of secretory glands.

Epidemiology: it most commonly appears in individuals aged 50-60 years. It is not a common disorder. Paget's disease of the nipple represents about 3% of mammary carcinomas and is more frequent in female patients; EMPD is a rare condition, with a male/female ratio of 2/1.

Clinical appearance: EMPD of the penis is first evident as a red, sometimes moist, well-demarcated patch that usually starts in the groins and then extends to the penis and scrotum; it may ulcerate. In some cases several multifocal patches develop, so that the penis, perineum and perianal area may be involved concurrently.

Clinical course: it may extend over a period of 10-15 years without evidence of invasive cancer or metastases. In a minority of patients, tumor cells infiltrate the dermis, adnexa, or lymph nodes. It may be associated with underlying malignancy of the urethra, ureter, bladder, prostate, or lower gastrointestinal tract. Recurrences are common, possibly because of a multicentric origin. The prognosis depends on the presence and type of the underlying malignancy, if any.

Diagnosis: it is established by histopathology characterized by the presence of large basophilic or vacuolated (Paget) cells in the epidermis.

Therapy: it consists of surgical excision that is radically complete into detection and ablation of underlying apocrine carcinoma, if present. Other options are excision by carbon dioxide laser therapy, radiation, or Mohs surgery. Radiotherapy has also been recommended as palliative treatment and can also be considered in patients who are not surgical candidates. Because this tumor tends to metastasize, regional lymph node evaluation is indicated. Topical chemotherapy with 5-fluorouracil and bleomycin has been tried, but it has provided only symptomatic relief.

Suggested Reading

Ekwueme KC, Zakhour HD, Parr NJ (2009) Extramammary Paget's disease of the penis: a case report and review of the literature. J Med Case Rep 6:3-4

Kariya K, Tsuji T, Schwartz RA (2004) Trial of low dose 5-fluorouracil/cisplatin therapy for advanced extramammary Paget's disease. Dermatol Surg 30:328-331

Kitajima S, Yamamoto K, Tsuji T, Schwartz RA (1997) Triple extramammary Paget's disease. Dermatol Surg 23:1035-8

Li B, Ding Q (2011) Extramammary Paget's disease involving the penis, scrotum and the axilla. Australas J Dermatol 52:18-20

Renaud-Vilmer C, Cavelier-Balloy B, Boazec L et al (2012) Metastatic extramammary Paget's disease of the scrotum. Ann Dermatol Venereol 139:387-90

Sandhu N, Schwartz RA (2012) Paget disease, extramammary. eMedicine from WebMD. Updated 2011. Available at http://emedicine.medscape.com/article/1100397-overview

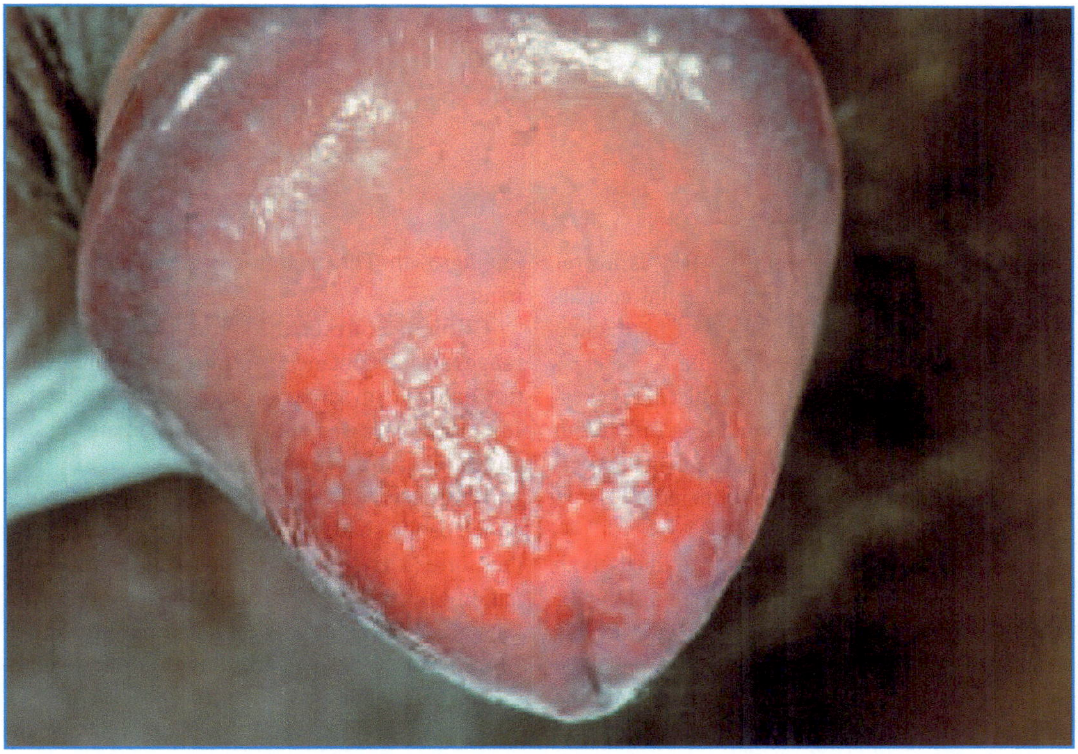

Fig. 8.7 Erythematous, oozing, and slightly infiltrated plaque on the glans

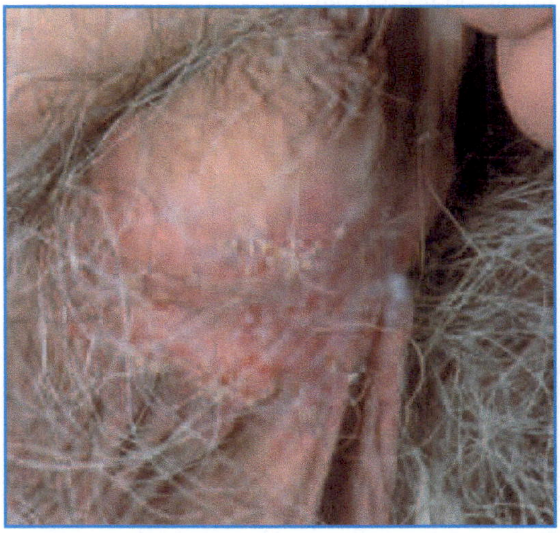

Fig. 8.8 Erythematous and scaling plaque on the shaft

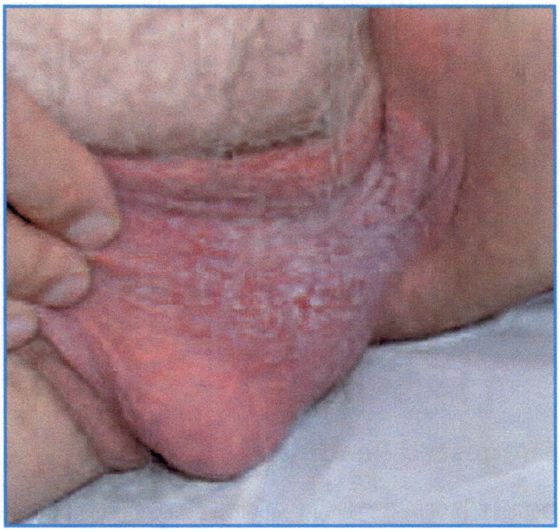

Fig. 8.9 Reddish and scaling plaque on the scrotum

In Situ Carcinomas

Bowenoid Papulosis

Definition: Bowenoid Papulosis (BP) is a precancerous skin condition (intraepithelial neoplasia) characterized by the presence of pigmented verrucous papules on the genital area.

Etiology: BP is an HPV-related disease, generally associated with HPV-16 and less often with HPV-18 and -33 infection. Because of its association with HPV, this disorder is considered a sexually transmitted disease.

Epidemiology: it affects young individuals, both males and females. It is more frequent in immunocompromised patients, such as HIV-infected people. It can occur anywhere in the anogenital skin, but the most frequent localizations are the penis and the vaginal labia.

Clinical appearance: it is characterized by skin-colored or pigmented papules, 2-20 mm in diameter, localized anywhere in the anogenital area, especially on the penile shaft or the perineum; these lesions can be isolated or grouped, with smooth or verrucous surfaces, sometimes showing rapid growth. The condition is generally asymptomatic.

Clinical course: the natural history of BP ranges from spontaneous remission to rare evolution into an invasive squamous cell carcinoma. Immunosuppressed patients are at greater risk of developing invasive carcinomas.

Diagnosis: the presence of pigmented papules on the penile shaft of a young man should point to the correct diagnosis. Histopathological examination is mandatory for diagnosis. It shows cellular and architectural atypia, similar to that of Bowen's disease. Evidence of tumor invasion into the underlying dermis is absent.

Therapy: it involves destruction of the lesions by medical and/or surgical intervention, such as topical 5-fluorouracil or imiquimod, cryotherapy, diathermy, laser therapy or surgical excision. Spontaneous regression occasionally occurs. Although BP appears to be a benign condition, close follow-up is essential.

Suggested Reading

Dehen L (1999) Bowenoid papulosis. Ann Dermatol Venereol 126:267-9

Matuszewski M, Michajłowski I, Michajłowski J et al (2009) Topical treatment of bowenoid papulosis of the penis with imiquimod. J Eur Acad Dermatol Venereol 23:978-9

Papadopoulos AJ, Schwartz RA, Janniger CK (2000) Bowenoid papulosis. Dermatol Klin (Wroclaw) 2: 91-3

Papadopoulos AJ, Schwartz RA, Lefkowitz A et al (2002) Extragenital bowenoid papulosis associated with atypical human papillomavirus genotypes. J Cutan Med Surg 6:117-121.

Shastry V, Betkerur J, Kushalappa PA (2009) Bowenoid papulosis of the genitalia successfully treated with topical tazarotene: a report of two cases. Indian J Dermatol 54:283-6

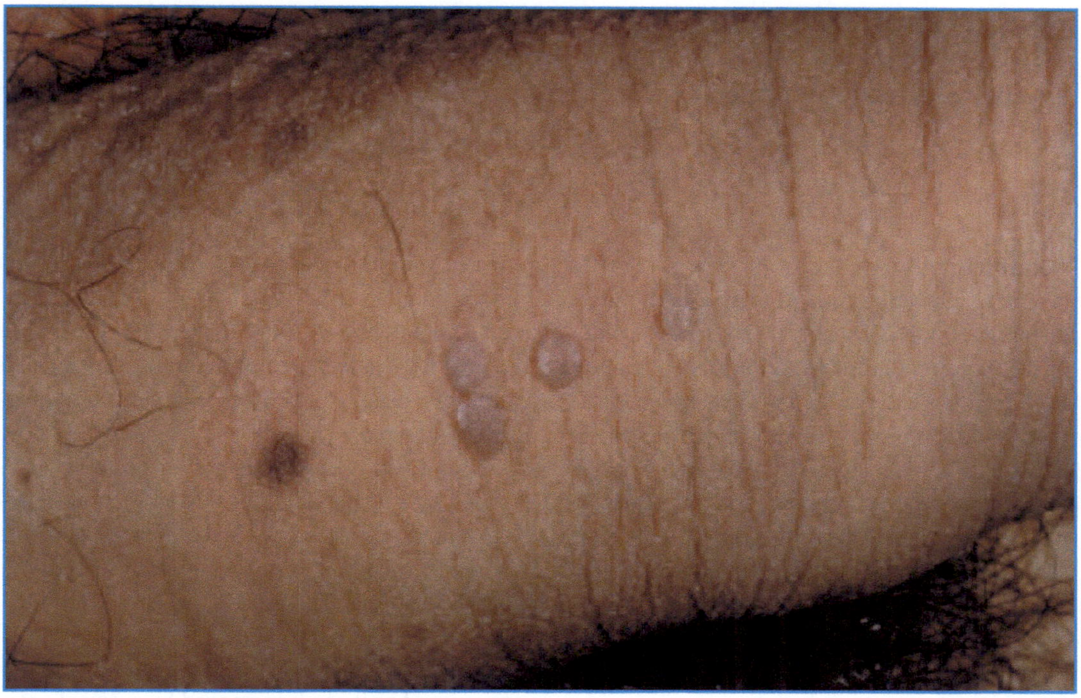

Fig. 8.10 Skin-colored and flat-topped papules on the shaft

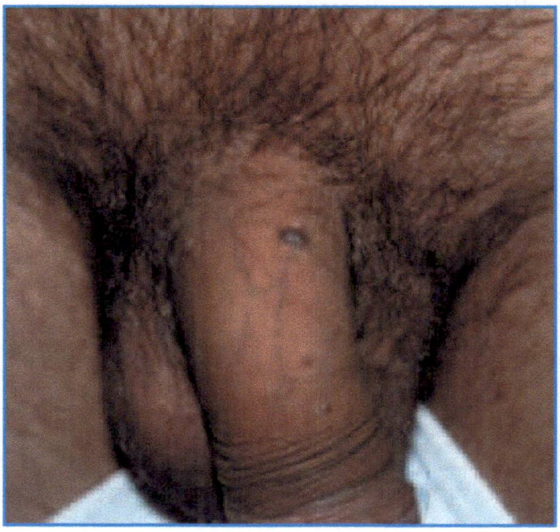

Fig. 8.11 Dark brown papules on the shaft

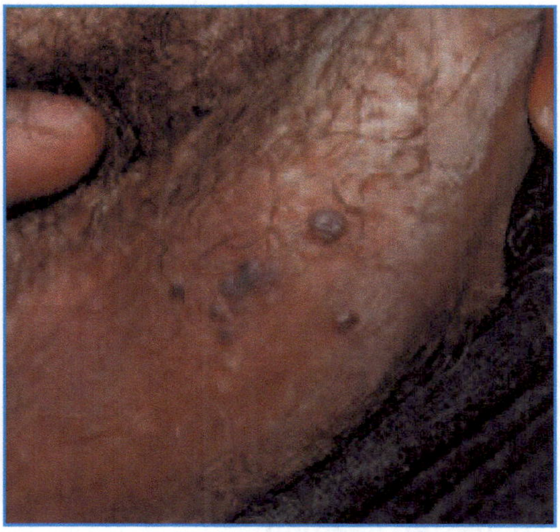

Fig. 8.12 Dark brown papules on the scrotum

In Situ Carcinomas

Erythroplasia of Queyrat

Definition: Erythroplasia of Queyrat (EQ) is a premalignant condition of the visible mucous membranes. It is considered to be Bowen's disease of the glans and prepuce and it is an intraepithelial squamous cell carcinoma (carcinoma in situ).

Etiology: it is not well known, but chronic irritative triggers are believed to play an important role. Circumcision may protect against the development of this disease, possibly because it facilitates better hygiene, with less accumulation of smegma, and reduced risk of chronic infection. EQ is virtually unknown in those circumcised early in infancy.

Epidemiology: it mostly affects middle-aged and older uncircumcised men.

Clinical appearance: it is characterized by a single erythematous patch, with a clear-cut border and lucent surface. It is asymptomatic and shows slow growth. It is generally localized on glans penis or inner foreskin. Lesions are often present for months to years before clinical attention is sought.

Clinical course: if not treated, EQ evolves in an invasive squamous cell carcinoma. Erosion and ulceration usually herald the development of invasive carcinoma.

Diagnosis: clinical suspicion must be confirmed by a histopathological examination showing atypical keratinocytes and numerous mitoses. Evidence of tumor invasion into the underlying dermis is absent. The most important differential diagnosis is Zoon's balanitis.

Therapy: the lesion can be treated with topical imiquimod or it can be removed by surgical excision, Mohs micrographic surgery, diathermy, laser therapy or photodynamic therapy. Circumcision is recommended for all patients because it eliminates the mucosal surface of the prepuce. Close follow-up is indicated.

Suggested Reading

Divakaruni AK, Rao AV, Mahabir B (2008) Erythroplasia of Queyrat with Zoon's balanitis: a diagnostic dilemma. Int J STD AIDS 19:861-3

Feldmeyer L, Krausz-Enderlin V, Tondury B et al (2011) Methylaminolaevulinic acid photodynamic therapy in the treatment of erythroplasia of Queyrat. Dermatology 223:52-6

Micali G, Lacarrubba F, Dinotta F et al (2010) Treating skin cancer with topical cream. Expert Opin Pharmacother 11:1515-27

Micali G, Nasca MR, De Pasquale R (2006) Erythroplasia of Queyrat treated with imiquimod 5% cream. J Am Acad Dermatol 55:901-3

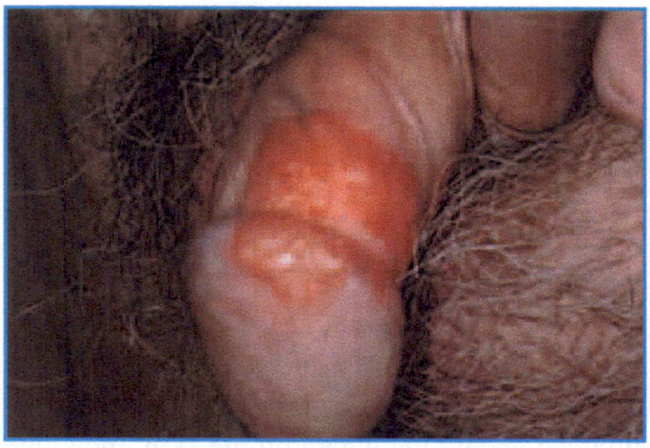

Fig. 8.13 Sharply marginated, glistening, and red patch involving the glans and foreskin

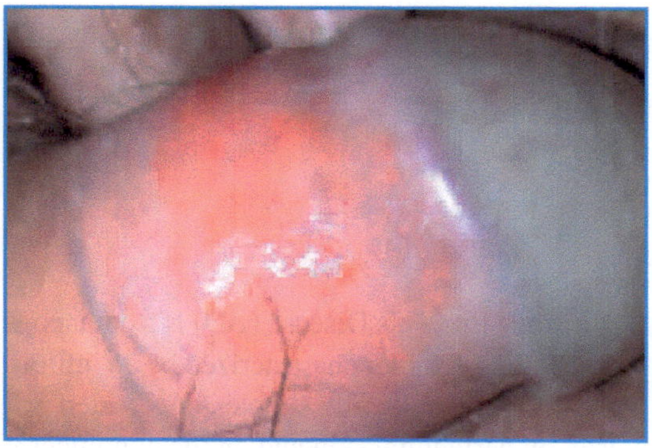

Fig. 8.14 Erythematous and oozing patch on the foreskin

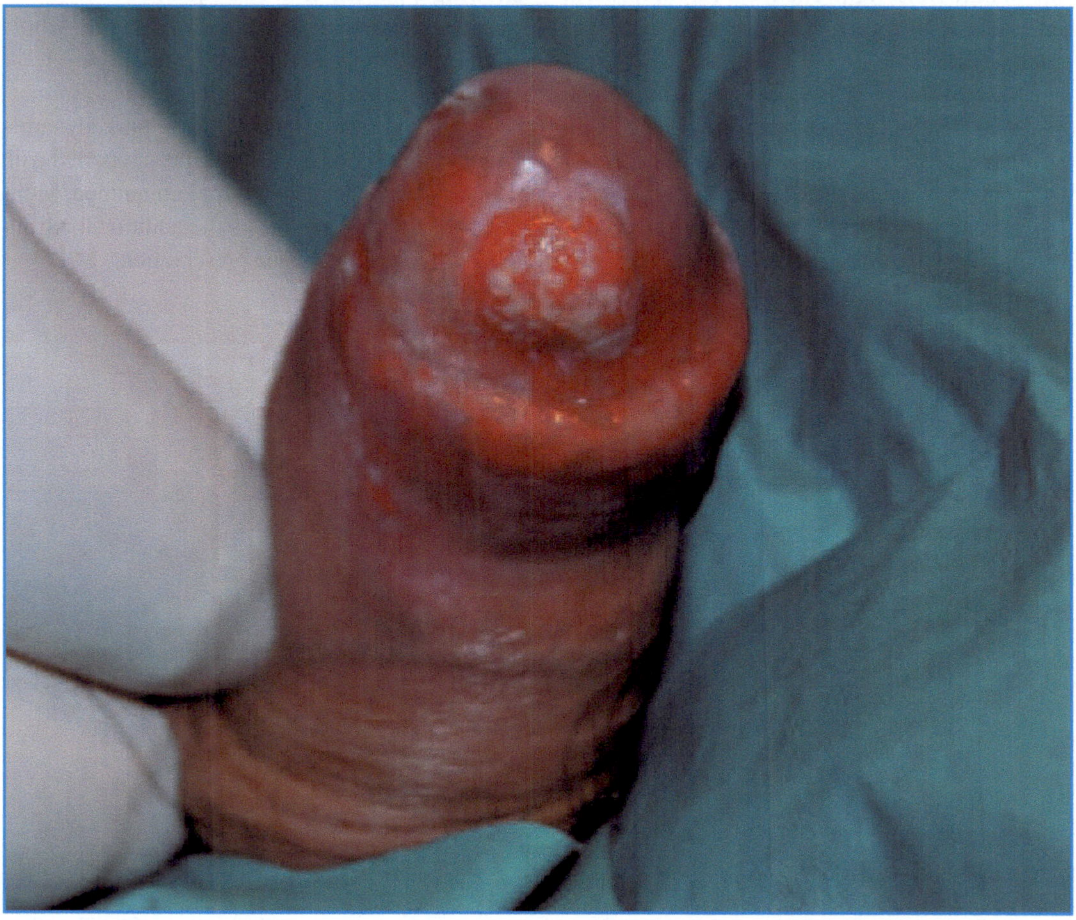

Fig. 8.15 Evolution towards invasive squamous cell carcinoma of the glans

In Situ Carcinomas

Bowen's Disease

Definition: Bowen's Disease (BD) is a cutaneous precancerous disorder characterized by an infiltrative and slowly enlarging skin lesion, located primarily on perigenital skin and on the nonmucosal side of the genitalia. It can be considered as an early stage or intraepidermal form of squamous cell carcinoma.

Etiology: it is not completely clear, but exposure to ultraviolet light, chemical carcinogens, arsenic, and HPV infections are considered important risk factors.

Epidemiology: it is a common dermatosis, generally affecting middle-aged and older patients. Bowen's disease is rarely encountered before the age of 50; most patients are aged over 60.

Clinical appearance: BD is characterized by a solitary, asymptomatic, gradually enlarging erythematous or erythematous-scaling plaque with an irregular border, variable size, and color ranging from light red to brownish-red; this kind of lesion can appear anywhere on the skin, including the penis.

Clinical course: if not treated, BD evolves into invasive squamous cell carcinoma.

Diagnosis: histopathological examination, showing a pattern of in situ squamous cell carcinoma with atypical keratinocytes in the whole epidermis, is necessary for diagnosis.

Therapy: the lesion can be treated with surgical excision, cryotherapy, diathermy or photodynamic therapy; some good results have been reported with topical 5-fluorouracil and topical imiquimod. Mohs micrographic surgery offers the additional advantage of maximizing tissue preservation.

Suggested Reading

Butani AK, Arbesfeld DM, Schwartz RA (2005) Premalignant and early squamous cell carcinoma. Clin Plast Surg 32:223-35

Shimizu A, Tamura A, Abe M et al (2012) Human papillomavirus type 56-associated Bowen's disease. Br J Dermatol 167:1161-4

Taliaferro SJ, Cohen GF (2008) Bowen's disease of the penis treated with topical imiquimod 5% cream. J Drugs Dermatol 7:483-5

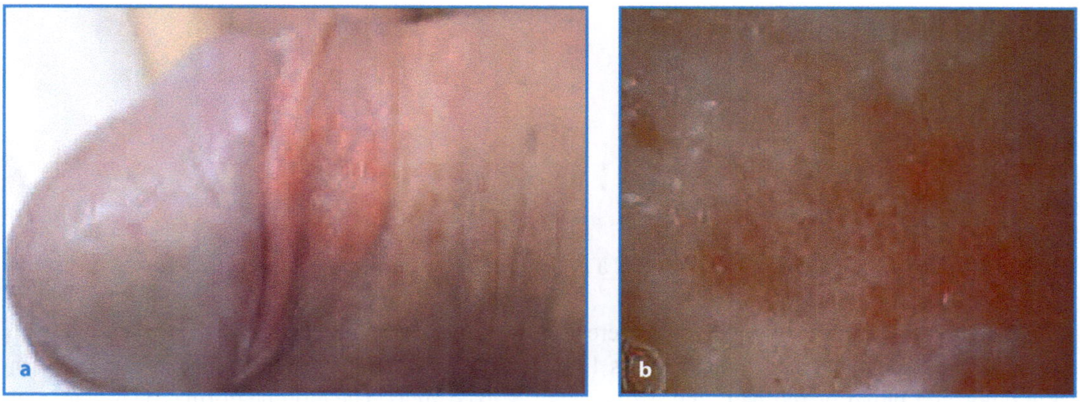

Fig. 8.16 a Erythematous, roundish, and solitary plaque on the foreskin. b Videodermatoscopy (X20) showing the presence of glomerular vessels and a scaly surface

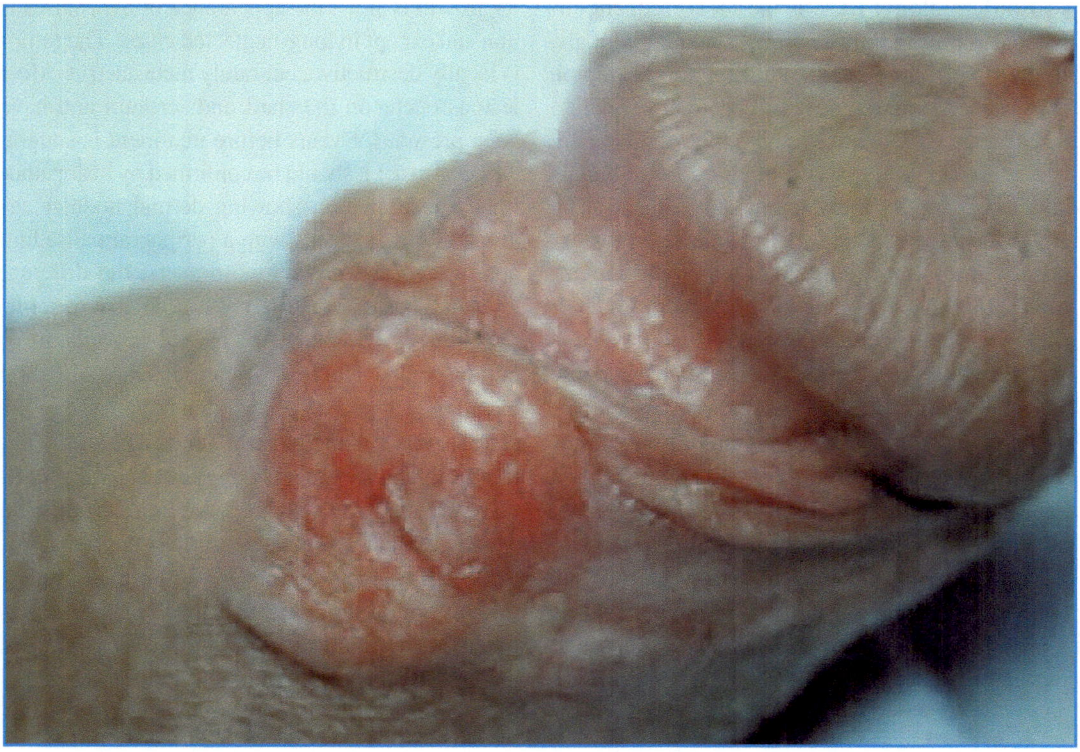

Fig. 8.17 Evolution towards invasive squamous cell carcinoma of the foreskin

Invasive Carcinomas

Basal Cell Carcinoma

Definition: Basal Cell Carcinoma (BCC) is a malignant skin tumor.

Etiology: it is a multifactorial disease; there are physical predisposing conditions, such as light skin color and blond or red hair, and exogenous risk factors, such as exposure to ultraviolet light, ionizing radiations, and arsenic ingestion. Some genodermatoses are also associated with a higher incidence of BCC, such as albinism, xeroderma pigmentosum, and the basal cell nevus syndrome.

Epidemiology: BCC is the most frequent cutaneous tumor in light-complexioned individuals. In the USA more than one million nonmelanoma skin cancers are diagnosed every year, of which 80-90% are BCC. It affects both men and women, it is more often diagnosed in elderly individuals and it is generally localized in sun-exposed skin. Given the low incidence of ultraviolet radiation exposure in the male genitalia, tumors are uncommon at this site. The male to female ratio for BCC of the genitalia appears to be about 1:4.

Clinical appearance: on the penis and the scrotum, BCC presents as a solitary skin-colored nodule 1 to 2 cm in diameter, generally asymptomatic. The lesion is smooth-surfaced, with a pearly translucent quality. There are different clinical variants of BCC, the most frequent being the nodular, superficial and morpheaform. The nodular type is the most common and presents as round, flesh-colored papule with telangiectases. It frequently ulcerates centrally, leaving a raised, pearly border with telangiectases. The superficial type presents as an erythematous or erythemato-scaling plaque or nodule, with a raised border; it can be multicentric, with areas of clinically normal skin intervening between clinically involved areas. The morpheaform type is characterized by proliferation of fibroblasts within the dermis and increased collagen deposition; it appears as a fibrotic, whitish sclerotic plaque that rarely ulcerates.

Clinical course: BCC is a malignant tumor, but its growth is slow; the appearance of metastases is unusual except in long-neglected cases. The tumor is locally destructive, but rarely metastasizes. Most lesions occur on the shaft and scrotum and have been present for years before treatment is sought.

Diagnosis: it should be confirmed by histopathological examination showing dermal nodular aggregates of basal cells with a peripheral palisading appearance and retraction artefacts; the different clinical types reflect different histological patterns.

Therapy: treatment of choice is excision or curettage and electrodessication. Depending on the clinical appearance, the number and size of the lesions, the age and general conditions of the patient, surgical treatments (surgical excision, curettage and electrodessication, Mohs micrographic surgery, diathermy, and cryosurgery) or nonsurgical treatments (imiquimod, 5-fluorouracil, radiotherapy, photodynamic therapy) can be implemented. For small lesions, complete excision of the tumor is generally curative. Incomplete treatment often results in local recurrence.

Suggested Reading

Gibson GE, Ahmed I (2001) Perianal and genital basal cell carcinoma: A clinicopathologic review of 51 cases. J Am Acad Dermatol 45:68-71

Lidder S, Lang KJ, Nakhdjevani A (2011) Basal cell carcinoma of the penis. Singapore Med J 52:201-2

Ribuffo D, Alfano C, Ferrazzoli PS et al (2002) Basal cell carcinoma of the penis and scrotum with cutaneous metastases. Scand J Plast Reconstr Surg Hand Surg 36:180-2

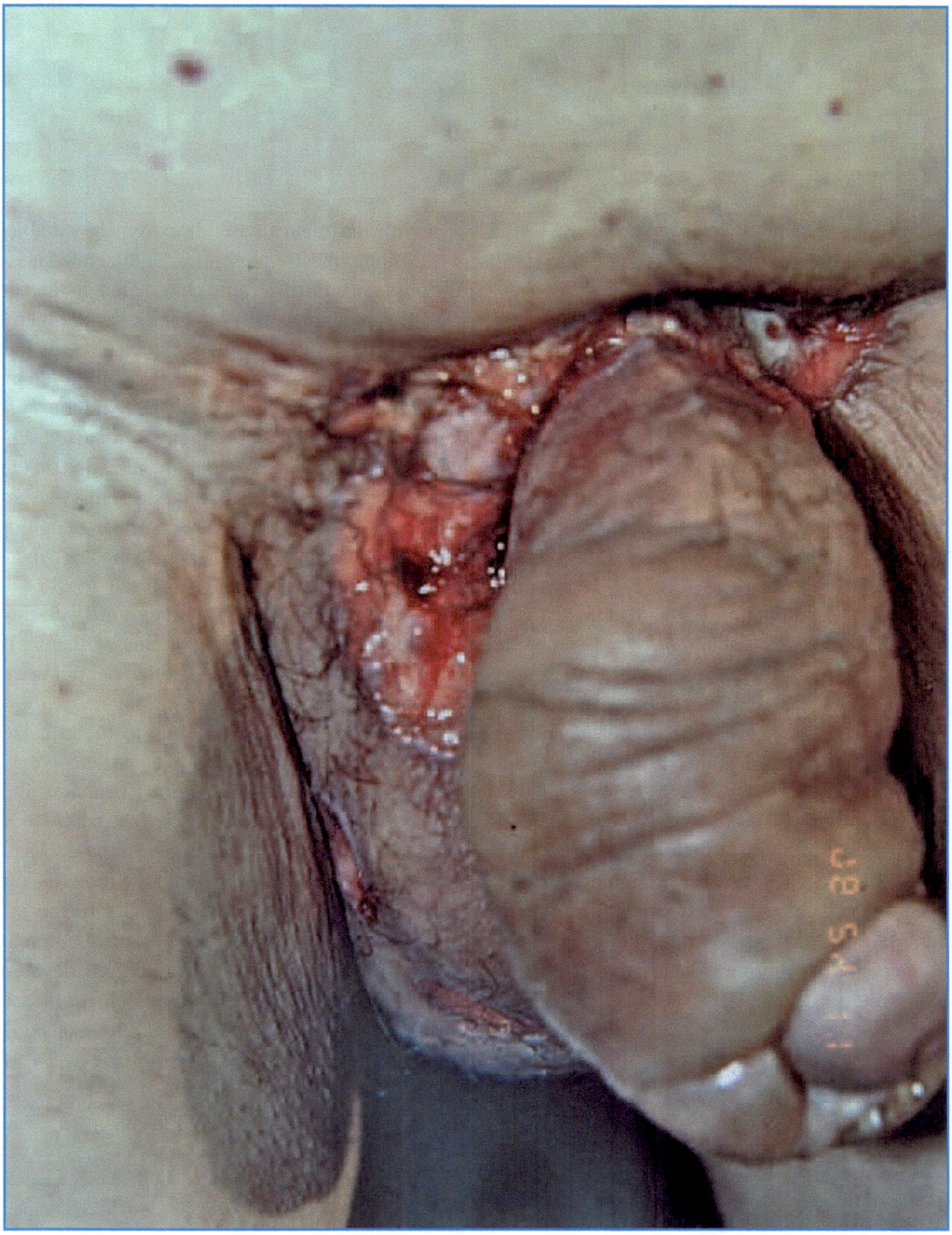

Fig. 8.18 Locally advanced and ulcerated tumor involving the pubis and the scrotum, associated with marked penile edema

Invasive Carcinomas

Squamous Cell Carcinoma

Definition: Squamous Cell Carcinoma (SCC) is a malignant tumor of the epidermal keratinocytes. It may be limited to the epidermal layer only (erythroplasia of Queyrat, Bowen's disease), or may invade into the deeper layers (invasive squamous cell carcinoma).

Etiology: it is unclear. SCC of the penis has been associated with phimosis. Most cases occur in elderly uncircumcised men. It is believed that the crucial factor is the link between foreskin retention and poor hygiene, and subsequent chronic balanitis. HPV infection (types 16 and 18, as well as 6, 11, and 30) is associated with 15-71% of penile squamous cell carcinomas. Other risk factors associated with the development of penile carcinoma include immunosuppression (transplant patients and HIV-infected individuals), and dermatological diseases such as lichen sclerosus and lichen planus. SCC of the scrotum has recently been related to PUVA therapy.

Epidemiology: although it is rare in persons younger than 40 years, the age at presentation ranges from 20-90 years. In the United States, penile cancer accounts for less than 1% of all malignancies. It is the most common malignant tumor of the penis, accounting for more than 95% of all malignant penile neoplasms. Scrotal SCC is much rarer, with fewer than 10 new cases reported annually in the United States.

Clinical appearance: it is extremely variable. The lesion typically presents as an ulcerated nodule or plaque one to several centimeters in diameter, often bleeding easily, and can exhibit either a flat or an exophytic, papillary clinical growth pattern. Most lesions present on the glans, followed by the prepuce and the coronal sulcus. Symptoms often include penile pain, malignant priapism, discharge, and difficulty voiding. Localization on the scrotum is also possible, usually as a solitary lesion that initially appears as a slowly growing papillomatous or wart-like nodule, or as an area of hyperkeratosis. Lymphadenopathy is present in 28-64% of cases at presentation. Most tumors are well-differentiated squamous cell carcinomas. Other variants include basaloid, sarcomatoid (or spindled), and verrucous growth patterns.

Clinical course: SCC tends to metastasize early to regional lymph nodes. The prognosis correlates with the extent of tumor invasion and lymph node status, because SCC of the penis tends to be a locally advanced, aggressive disease. Death typically occurs within 2 years if the tumor is left untreated. Nodal metastases, usually to the inguinal and/or iliac nodes, are the most common route of dissemination. Of note, 5-15% develop second primary lesions, often located in the residua of the penis. Complications are usually due to recurrence, which occurs in as many as 7% of

Suggested Reading

Bethune G, Campbell J, Rocker A et al (2012) Clinical and pathologic factors of prognostic significance in penile squamous cell carcinoma in a North American population. Urology 79:1092-7

Deem S, Keane T, Bhavsar R, El-Zawahary A et al (2011) Contemporary diagnosis and management of squamous cell carcinoma (SCC) of the penis. BJU Int 108:1378-92

Ferrándiz-Pulido C, de Torres I, García-Patos V (2012) Penile squamous cell carcinoma. Actas Dermosifiliogr 103:478-87

Micali G, Nasca MR, Innocenzi D, Schwartz RA (2006) Penile squamous cell carcinoma. J Am Acad Dermatol 54: 369-91

patients. In addition to the extent of tumor invasion and lymph node status, histologic type plays a role in prognosis. Worse prognosis is associated with basaloid and sarcomatoid subtypes. Enlargement of the inguinal nodes presents the same problem in scrotal cancer as in penile carcinoma.

Diagnosis: given the anatomic location and clinical presentation, the diagnosis of SCC is generally straightforward. Biopsy is necessary for a definitive diagnosis. Histopathology shows features of invasive carcinoma and can exhibit morphologic heterogeneity. The TNM system classifies cases into stages I-IV based on the extension of the tumor. Histologic grading using the modified Broder classification divides tumors into 4 histologic grades ranging from well-differentiated to poorly differentiated. Of note, well-differentiated tumors metastasize to regional lymph nodes at a rate of 50%, while moderately or poorly differentiated tumors have an 80-100% nodal metastatic rate. Hematogenous metastasis is uncommon, accounting for fewer than 2% of cases at diagnosis. One third of the cases metastasize early, so any suspicious lesion should be biopsied immediately and treatment instituted before metastasis or locally advanced disease occurs.

Therapy: the primary treatment for penile carcinoma is surgical. Surgical intervention involves wide excision, partial penectomy, or total penectomy. Excision of scrotal SCC requires at least 2cm margins with resection of the skin and underlying dartos muscle. The effectiveness of prophylactic bilateral inguinal node dissection is controversial. Sentinel lymph node biopsy has been successfully used in the surgical management of penile carcinoma, whereas the rarity of scrotal SCC makes it difficult to delineate definitive recommendations regarding node dissection. Radiation therapy has been employed with limited success in patients who are not surgical candidates. The role of chemotherapy, commonly utilizing cisplatin and bleomycin, is unclear. Combination chemotherapy and radiation using bleomycin-derived treatments have been successful in some cases, with response rates as high as 43%.

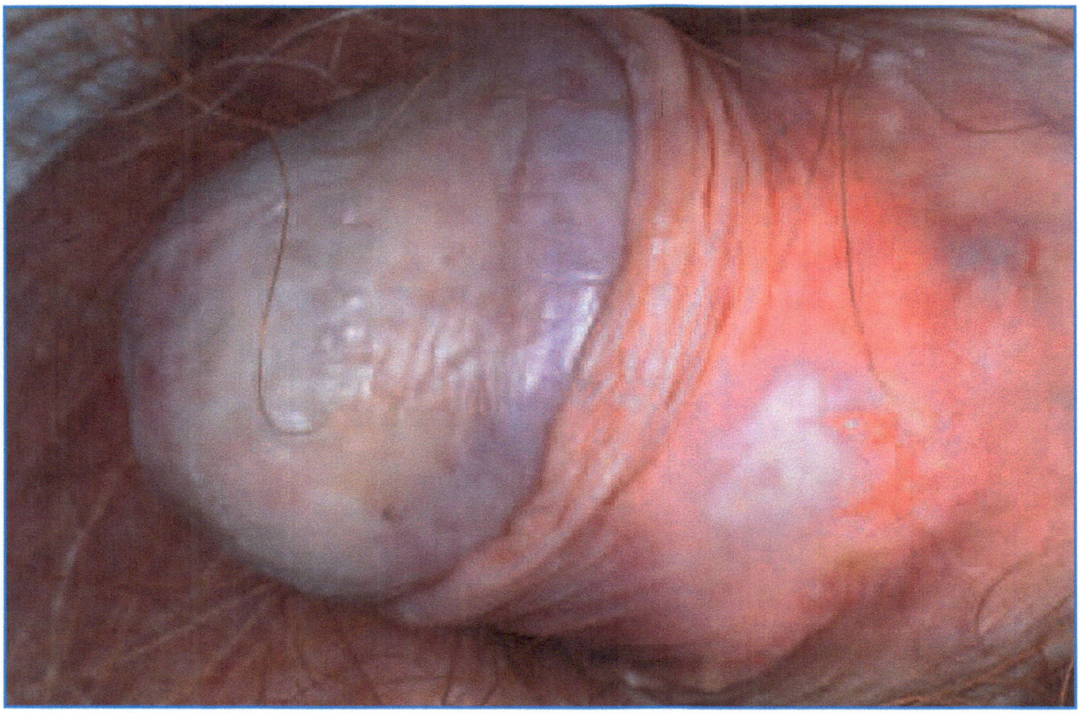

Fig. 8.19 Incipient and eroded nodule of the shaft

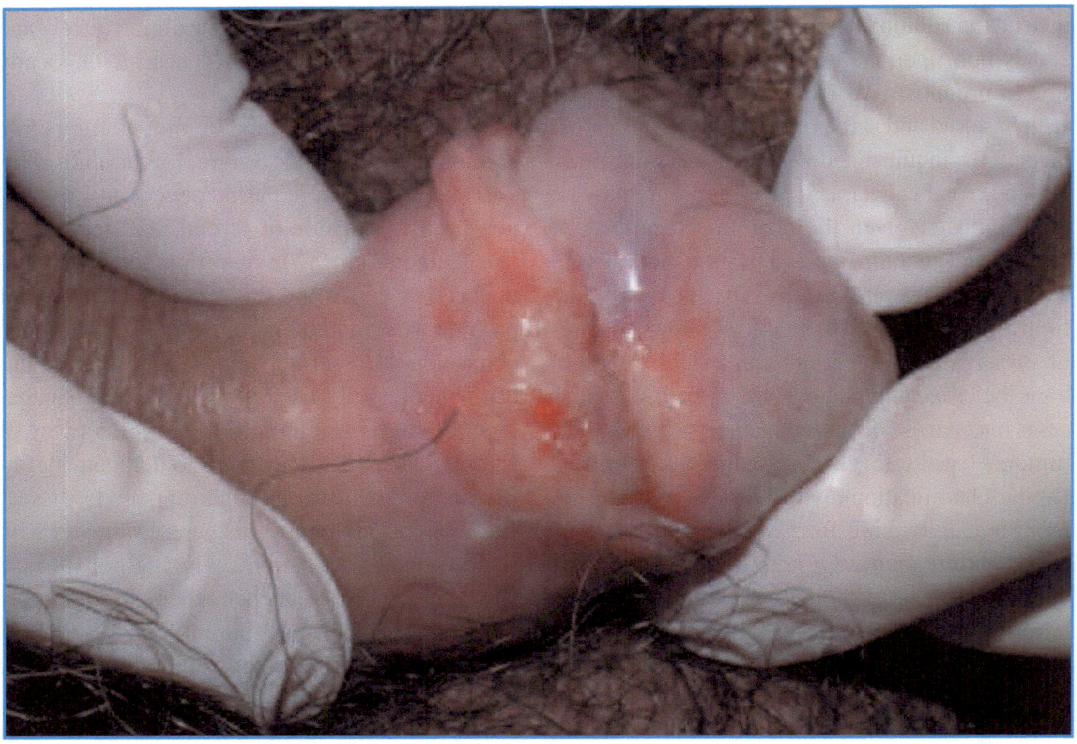

Fig. 8.20 Irregular, yellowish nodule, involving the glans, the coronal sulcus, and the foreskin

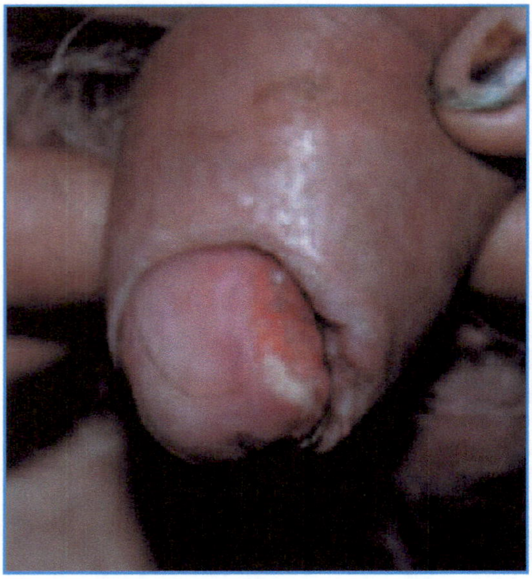

Fig. 8.21 Endophytic and ulcerative lesion on the glans

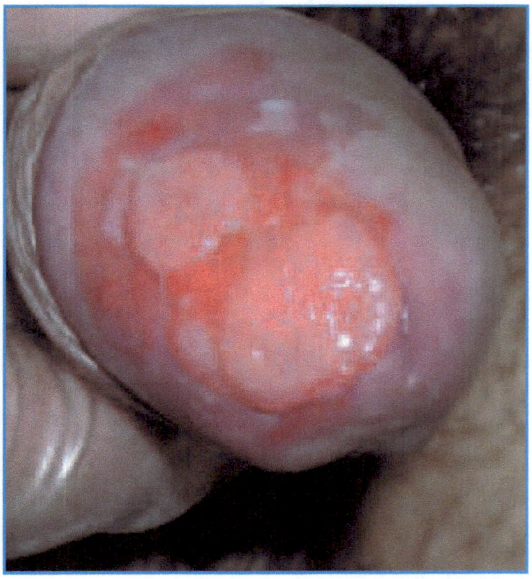

Fig. 8.22 Exophytic nodules on the glans

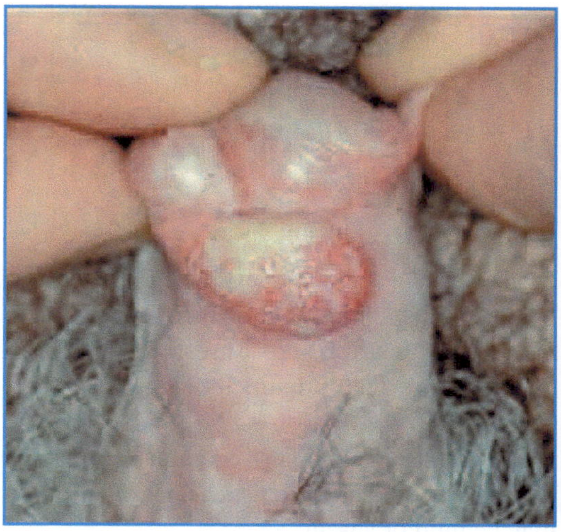

Fig. 8.23 Exophytic nodule on the foreskin

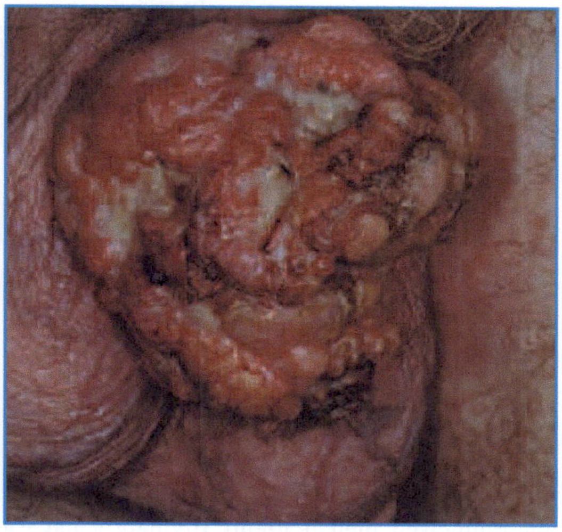

Fig. 8.24 Locally advanced and aggressive form in an HIV+ patient

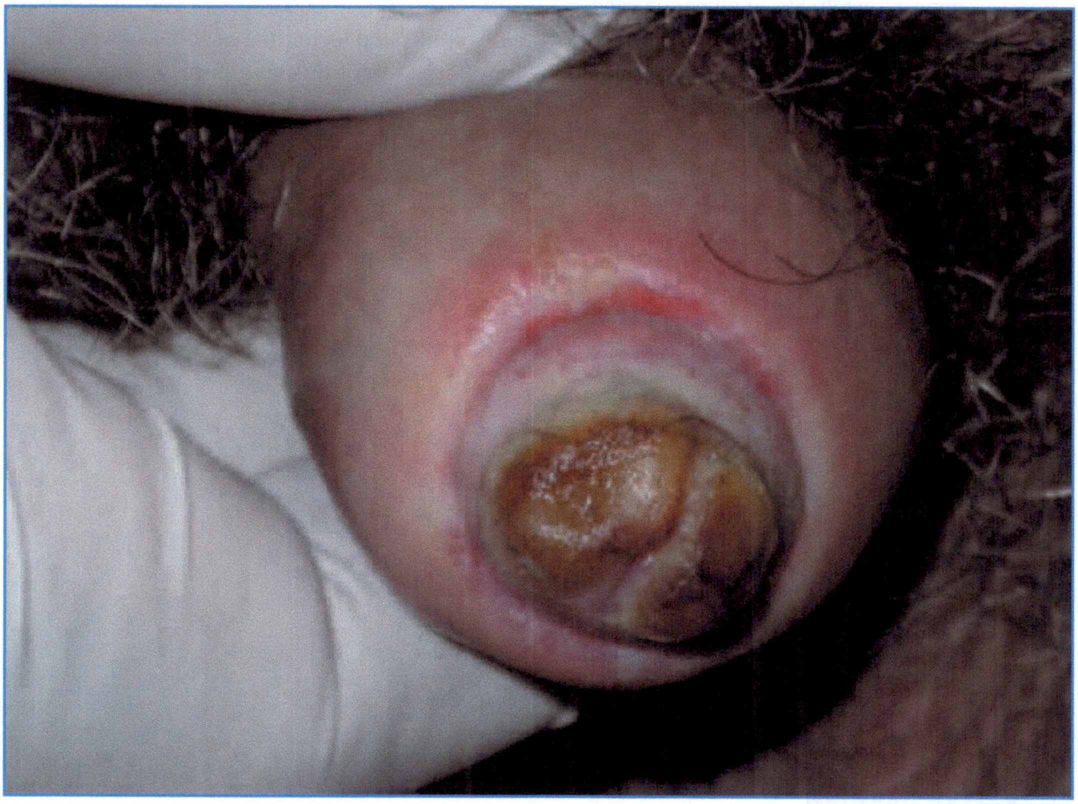

Fig. 8.25 Neoplastic phimosis

Invasive Carcinomas

Verrucous Carcinoma

Definition: Verrucous Carcinoma (VC) of the glans penis, commonly termed "giant condyloma acuminatum of Buschke and Loewenstein", represents a specific subtype of low-grade squamous cell carcinoma.

Etiology: it is often associated with HPV types 6 and 11. It is usually seen on the glans penis in uncircumcised men. Patients frequently have a history of balanitis, ulceration, or phimosis.

Epidemiology: it primarily affects men and generally occurs in patients aged 55-65 years. The majority of patients are uncircumcised men. It comprises approximately 5% of all penile cancers.

Clinical appearance: lesions are exophytic with a cauliflower-like appearance and they may occur on the glans and on the prepuce of uncircumcised individuals or on the anogenital mucosa.

Clinical course: it is well differentiated and rearely metastasizes, but it spreads aggressively by local extension and if left untreated it may destroy penile tissues entirely. Growth is characteristically locally invasive and destructive, and it has a tendency to extend proximally along the corpus urethrae.

Diagnosis: histological examination may be difficult, because characteristic neoplastic features may be mild or absent.

Therapy: the only satisfactory treatment is surgical ablation. Complete tumor extirpation should be performed at first presentation because VC can recur, become locally destructive, and, ultimately, cause death. The microscopically controlled technique of Mohs is well suited for extirpation of this neoplasm. Radiation therapy may predispose patients to metastatic disease. An extensive neoplastic process involving the shaft may require partial or complete phallectomy.

Suggested Reading

Chuanyu S, Ke X, Jie Z et al (2011) Surgical treatment for 11 cases of penile verrucous carcinoma. Ann Dermatol 23:346-9

Mokos I, Bukvi Mokos Z, Ljubojevi S et al (2012) Penile cutaneous horn ten years after treatment of verrucous squamous cell carcinoma on penile glans: case report. Acta Dermatovenerol Croat 20:30-3

Schwartz RA (1995) Verrucous carcinoma of the skin and mucosa. J Am Acad Dermatol 32:1-21

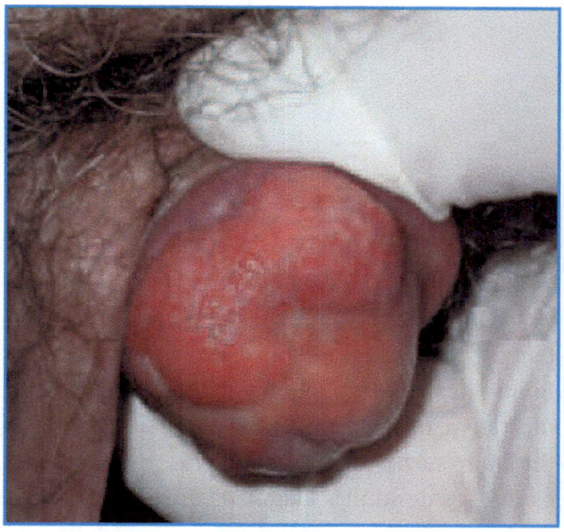

Fig. 8.26 Warty nodule on the glans

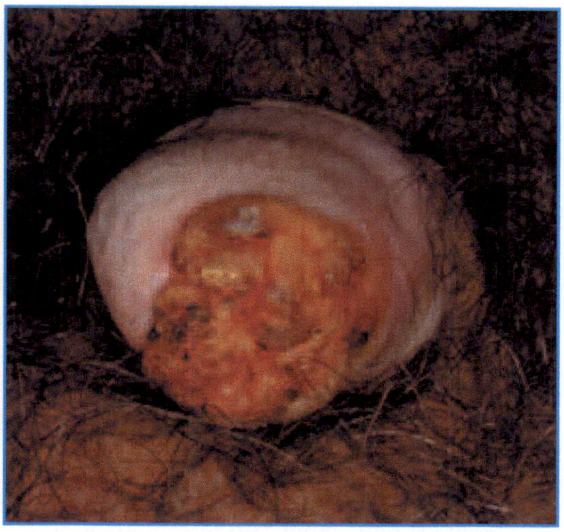

Fig. 8.27 Exophytic and warty mass on the glans

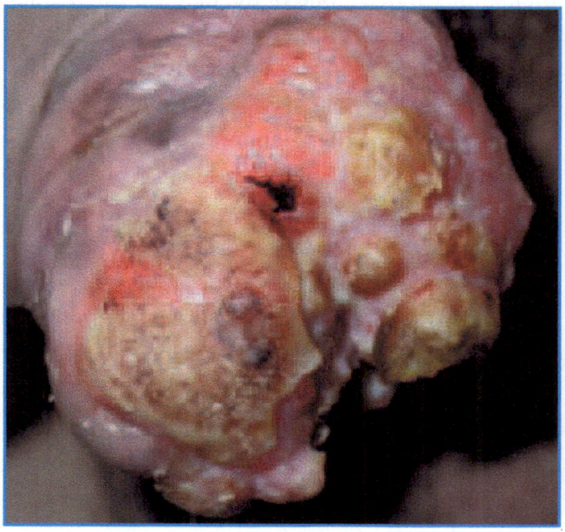

Fig. 8.28 Locally advanced and destructive bulk on the penis

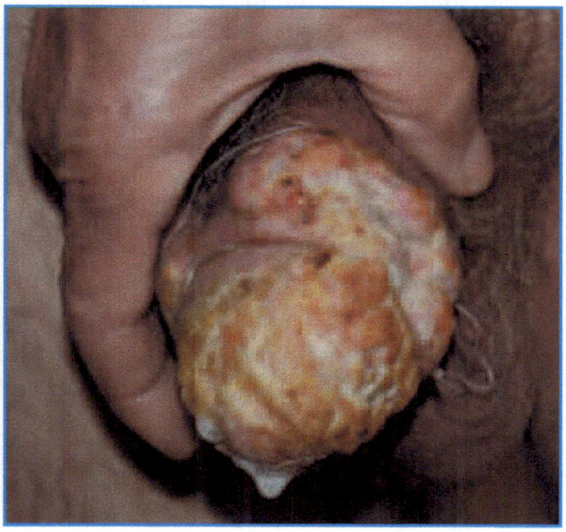

Fig. 8.29 Giant form of the penis

Melanoma

Definition: melanoma is an uncommon neoplasm of the male genitalia. Primary tumor sites include the penis, scrotum, and urethra.

Etiology: it is mostly related to genetic and environmental factors (unshielded UV exposure of genitalia).

Epidemiology: the incidence of primary penile melanoma is only about 1%; melanoma accounts for fewer than 2% of primary malignant tumors of the penis. Men aged 50-70 years are generally affected. On the penis, the most common tumor site is the glans (55% in one series); however, melanoma has been described on both the prepuce (28%) and the shaft (9%).

Clinical appearance: melanomas may vary in presentation from macules to papules and nodules, of varying color. The lesions are typically asymmetric macules with irregular borders and variable pigmentation. Clinically evident inguinal lymph node enlargement is seen in a minority of patients.

Clinical course: staging is based on the TNM classification, although the usual prognostic markers, such as the Breslow classification and Clark's level of anatomical invasion, which have been validated and applied to melanomas elsewhere, have not been validated in melanoma of the penis.

Diagnosis: penile melanomas are usually diagnosed late. Early diagnosis is of paramount importance because the risk of distant metastases is high. Physical examination is notable for a large, ulcerative, hemorrhagic, necrotic, lesion involving the entire surface of the glans penis. Biopsy is necessary for definitive diagnosis, histopathological examination demonstrating a generally ulceronecrotic surface and numerous atypical melanocytic cells. A problem in clinical practice is recognizing a pigmented penile lesion as a melanoma. Indeed, one of the major mimickers of mucosal melanoma, and thus of penile melanomas, is melanosis. Clinically, despite its benign behavior, melanosis can, at times, share features with malignant melanoma: asymmetry, irregular borders, multifocality, variegated pigmentary patterns and large size.

Therapy: surgical excision is the primary treatment for melanoma of the male genitalia. Partial penectomy with or without inguinal lymph node dissection is the most common surgical therapy for penile and urethral tumors. Wide local excision is used to treat scrotal tumors. Sentinel lymph node biopsy is performed in some cases. Adjuvant chemotherapy or radiotherapy can be used in more advanced cases.

Suggested Reading

De Giorgi V, Grazzini M, Massi D et al (2010) Melanoma of the penis: a clinical dermoscopic case study. Acta Derm Venereol 90:87-8

Dogu GG, Yaren A, Tuncay L et al (2012) Primary malignant melanoma of the penis: a case report. Med Oncol 29:1300-3

Johnson MH, Brandes SB, Humphrey PA (2012) Recurrent and metastatic malignant melanoma of the penis. J Urol 187:1438-9

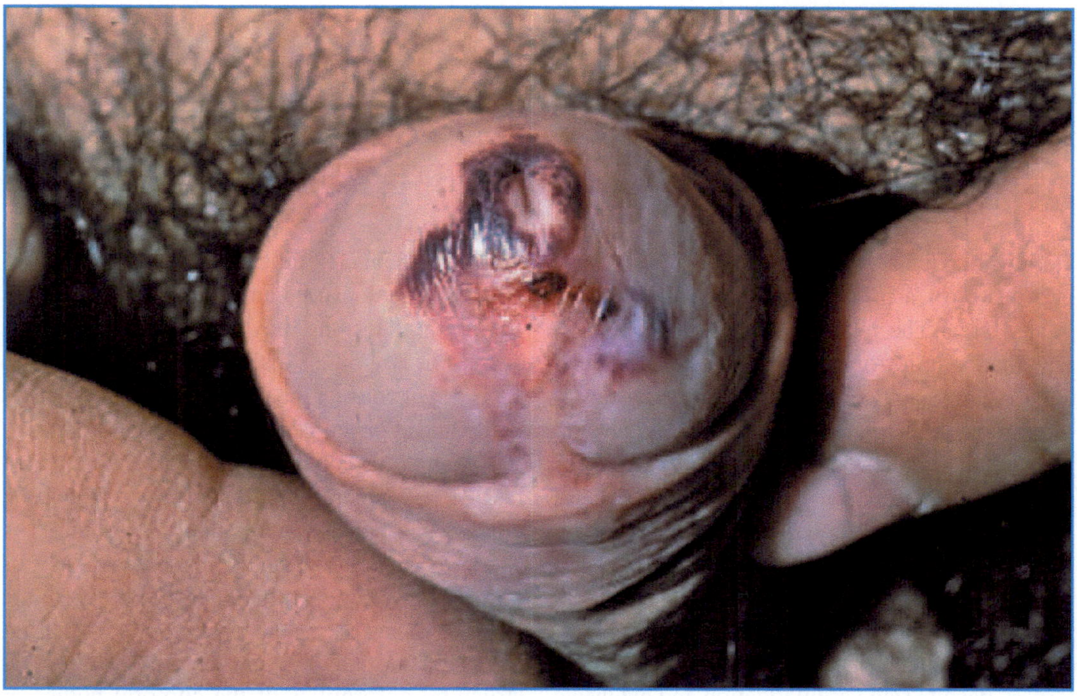

Fig. 8.30 Multicolored and irregular macule on the glans

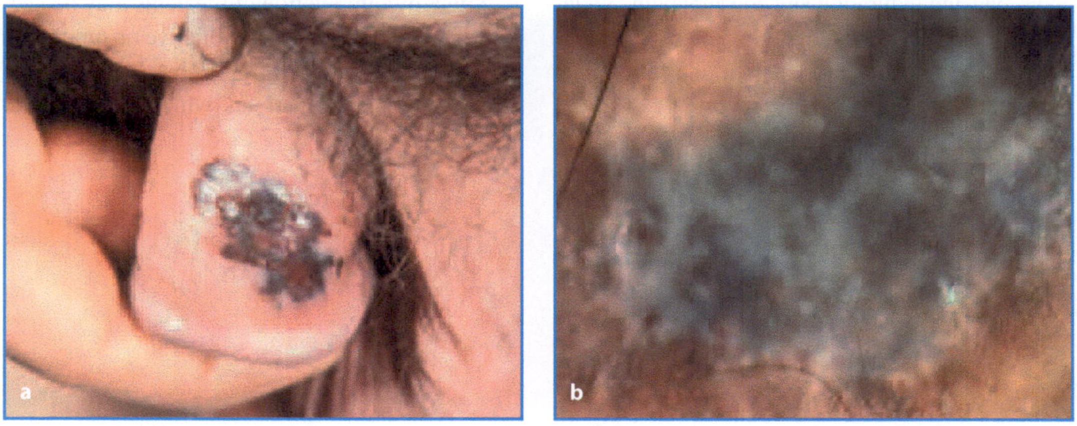

Fig. 8.31 a Multicolored and asymmetric macule on the penis with irregular borders. b Videodermatoscopy (X20) showing the presence of a grayish-blue veil

Cutaneous Metastatic Disease

Definition: Cutaneous Metastatic Disease (CMD) is a lesion of a primary tumor localized in the genital area. The majority of metastatic lesions take their origin from the neighboring genitourinary organs, mainly prostate and bladder. Metastatic lesions on the glans penis may rarely develop in patients with an underlying genitourinary or gastrointestinal carcinoma.

Etiology: it is the same as for the primary tumor.

Epidemiology: CMD is rare; the mean age at presentation of most tumors is between 60 and 80 years. Metastatic involvement of the penis is relatively infrequent, compared to its primary counterpart, despite rich vascularization and extensive circulatory communication between the penis and the neighboring organs.

Clinical appearance: the lesions may present as solitary nodules or they may infiltrate the entire penis, causing induration and constant pain. Nodular or ulcerative lesions involving the corpora cavernosa or priapism are the main modes of clinical presentation. Priapism may occur with varying frequencies, but it is a prominent feature in nearly 40% of patients. Nodules are the most likely lesions and demonstrate an inclination to ulcerate. Periurethral lesions may be confused with abscesses or Peyronie's disease.

Clinical course: the primary site in most cases is the bowel or the genitourinary tract. Penile involvement is usually associated with disseminated disease and generally portends a poor prognosis; death usually occurs in less than 12 months.

Diagnosis: it is usually made by biopsy or corporeal aspiration, which helps to differentiate between metastases and primary tumors. Metastatic lesions usually present as filling defects or structural deformities of the corporal bodies or glans. Noninvasive modalities are being increasingly used to stage the disease, such as color-coded duplex ultrasonography, computed tomography scan and magnetic resonance imaging.

Therapy: amputation of the penis may be necessary. In most cases, only palliative or supportive therapy is indicated. Surgical intervention may prove beneficial in patients with primary rectal carcinomas.

Suggested Reading

Chaux A, Amin M, Cubilla AL et al (2011) Metastatic tumors to the penis: a report of 17 cases and review of the literature. Int J Surg Pathol 19:597-606

Jones VS, Chandra S, Smile SR et al (2000) A unique case of metastatic penile basal cell carcinoma. Indian J Pathol Microbiol 43:465-6

Khandpur S, Reddy BS, Kaur H (2002) Multiple cutaneous metastases from carcinoma of the penis. J Dermatol 29:296-9

Schwartz RA (1995) Cutaneous metastatic disease. J Am Acad Dermatol 33:161-82

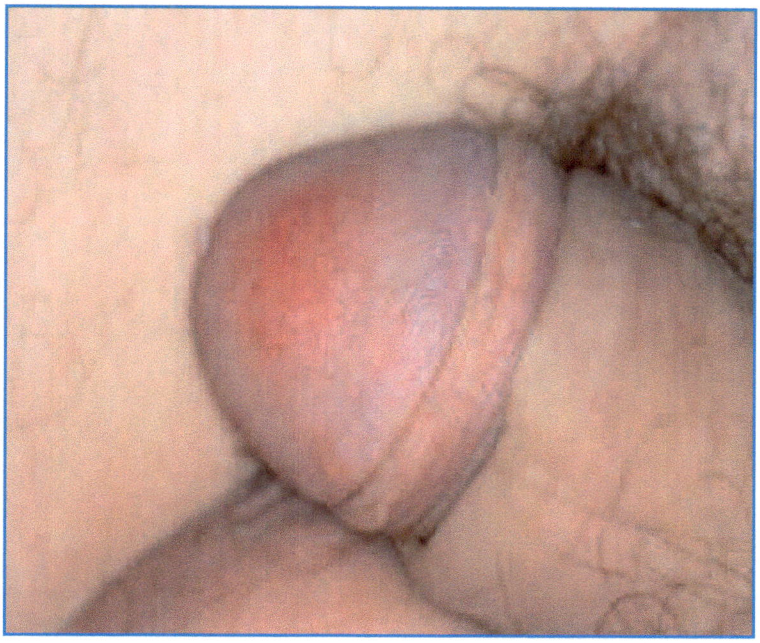

Fig. 8.32 Solitary red patch on the glans

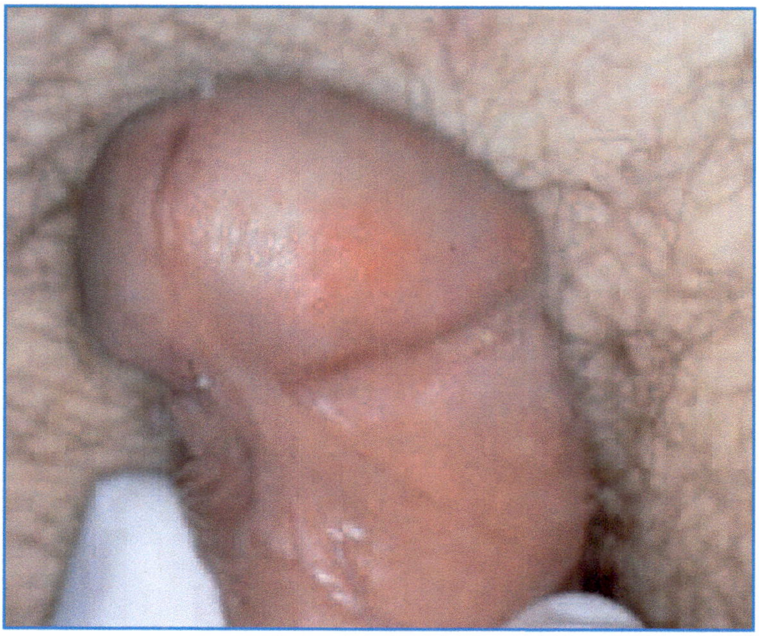

Fig. 8.33 Slight red patch on the glans

9 Dysembrioplastic Disorders

Pompeo Donofrio, Paola Donofrio, Maria Grazia Francia, and Maria Rita Nasca

P. Donofrio (✉)
School of Dermatology and Venereology
"Federico II" University of Naples, Naples, Italy
e-mail: dermodonofrio@hotmail.it

G. Micali et al., *Atlas of Male Genital Disorders*,
DOI: 10.1007/978-88-470-2787-9_9, © Springer-Verlag Italia 2013

Fordyce's Spots

Definition: Fordyce's Spots (FS) are ectopic sebaceous glands which appear on mucosal surfaces.

Etiology: the spots are a natural occurrence. They are not known to be associated with any disease and they are not infectious.

Epidemiology: FS are common in men of all ages.

Clinical appearance: small, painless, barely raised, smooth, yellow papules about 1 mm in diameter, that may appear on the scrotum and on the shaft of the penis and that are more evident when the mucosa is stretched. Sometimes they are so numerous that they appear as confluent patches. They are usually asymptomatic.

Clinical course: FS appear after puberty and persist indefinitely.

Diagnosis: it is made from clinical observation.

Therapy: since they are benign and asymptomatic, no treatment is necessary. Reassurance is all that is needed. Laser treatment, electric cautery or liquid nitrogen freezing can sometimes be used if FS are of aesthetic concern, but the patient must be warned of possible significant scarring.

Suggested Reading

Lee JH, Lee JH, Kwon NH et al (2012) Clinicopathologic manifestations of patients with Fordyce's spots. Ann Dermatol 24:103-6

Micali G, Lacarrubba F (2011) Augmented diagnostic capability using videodermatoscopy on selected infectious and non-infectious penile growths. Int J Dermatol 50:1501-5

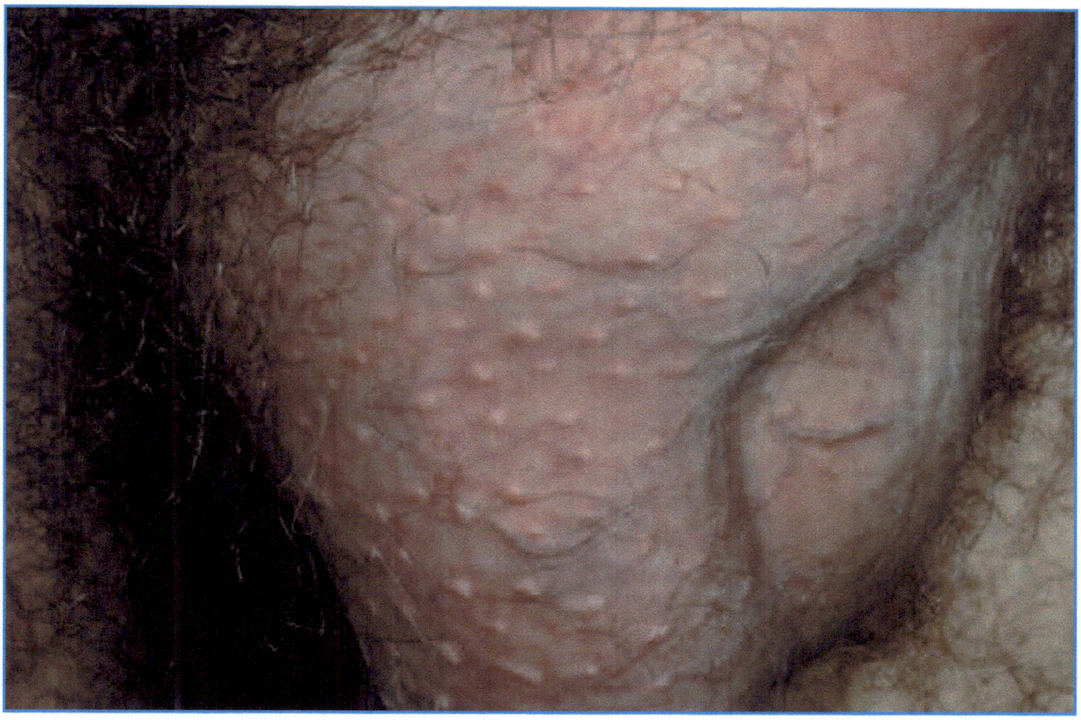

Fig. 9.1 Small, round, barely raised, and yellowish papules on the scrotum and proximal shaft

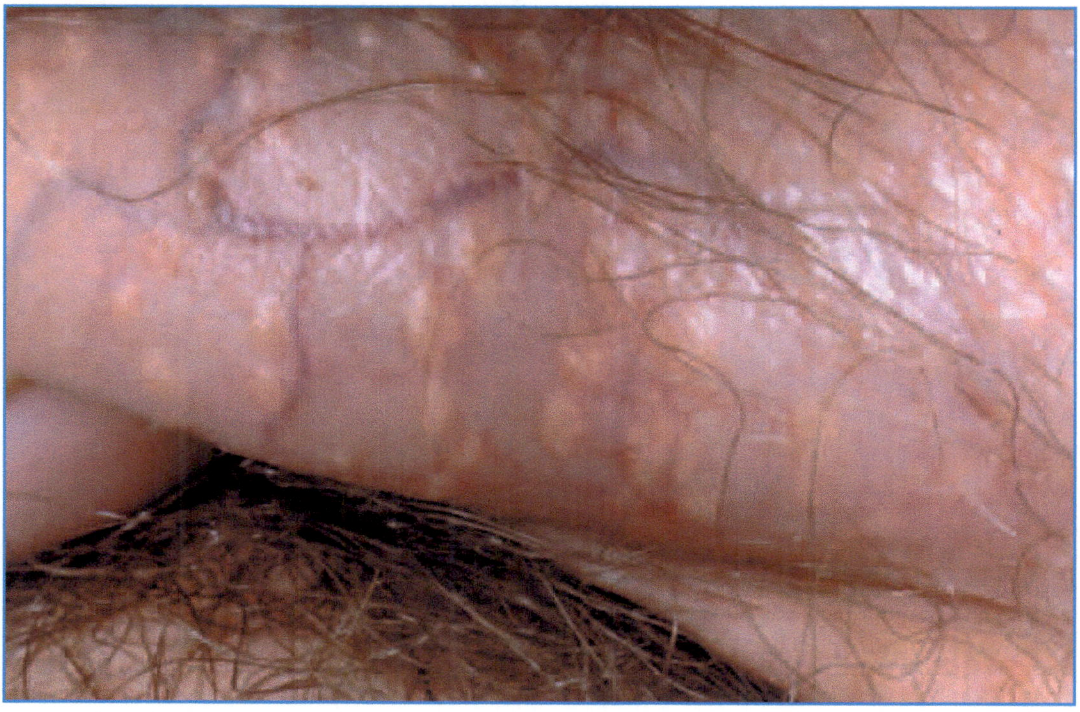

Fig. 9.2 Smooth and yellowish papules on the shaft

Sebaceous Hyperplasia

Definition: Sebaceous Hyperplasia (SH) is a proliferative abnormality of sebaceous glands. It is a common, benign condition that occurs as an appreciable enlargement of the pilosebaceous unit in nonectopic locations.

Etiology: higher sensitivity of the sebaceous cells to androgens, leading to an increase in cellular proliferation, may be a possible cause of penile SH. Inflammatory stimulation by CD8+ lymphocytes may also play a role.

Epidemiology: in contrast to facial lesions, the majority of penile SH cases seem to appear at an earlier age.

Clinical appearance: SH appears as single or multiple soft and asymptomatic papules, of less than 3 mm, which are skin-colored or yellowish. A small dimple representing the follicle outlet may be visible in the center of the larger lesions. Small numbers of sebaceous glands are commonly found anywhere on the shaft, but their concentration is noticeably increased in its proximal quarter.

Clinical course: SH persist indefinitely and it runs a benign course.

Diagnosis: it is typically clinical. Dermoscopy can aid in the differential diagnosis, showing a pattern characterized by aggregated yellowish-white-globules.

Therapy: SH is completely benign and does not require treatment. However, lesions can be cosmetically unfavorable and sometimes bothersome when irritated. Treatment is not necessary other than for cosmetic purposes. Current approaches include shave excision, bichloroacetic acid application, cryotherapy, carbon dioxide laser ablation, electrodessication, erbium or yttrium-aluminum-garnet laser ablation and pulsed-dye laser photothermolysis. Isotretinoin has also been used in some cases. The risk of permanent scarring must be considered. It is important to reassure the patient that SH is a benign and nontransmissible condition.

Suggested Reading

Ena P, Origa D, Massarelli G (2009) Sebaceous gland hyperplasia of the foreskin. Clin Exp Dermatol 34:372-4

Kim HS, Lee JY, Kim HO, Park YM (2011) Sebaceous hyperplasia of the scrotum and penile shaft. Ann Dermatol 23:S341-2

Niemann C (2009) Differentiation of the sebaceous gland. Dermatoendocrinol 1:64-7

Zampeli VA, Makrantonaki E, Tzellos T, Zouboulis CC (2012) New pharmaceutical concepts for sebaceous gland diseases: implementing today's pre-clinical data into tomorrow's daily clinical practice. Curr Pharm Biotechnol 13:1898-913

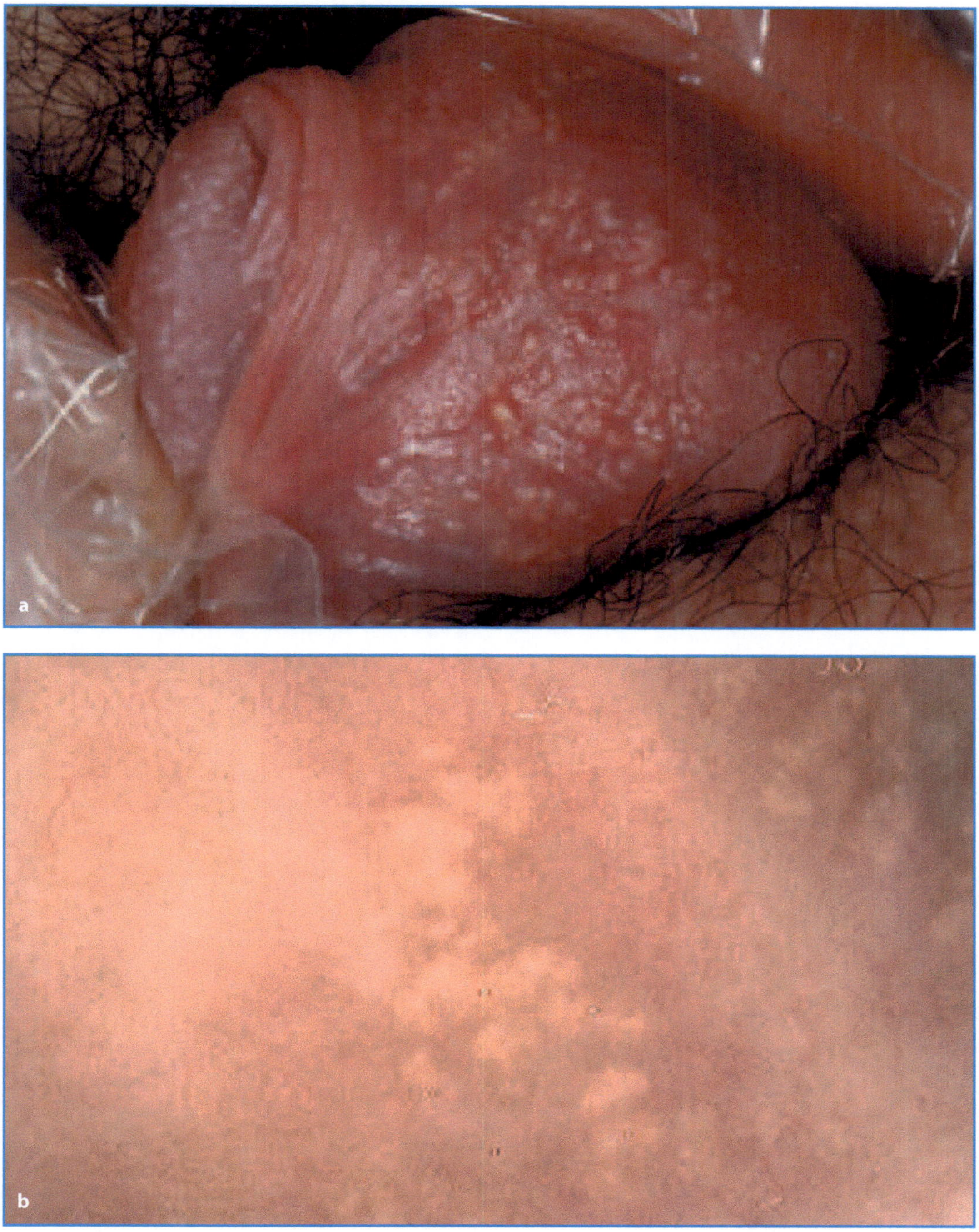

Fig. 9.3 a Grouped yellowish papules on the foreskin. **b** Videodermatoscopy (X20) showing a pattern composed of aggregated yellowish-white globules

Median Raphe Cysts

Definition: Median Raphe Cysts (MRC) are congenital epidermal cysts forming in the median penile raphe, which corresponds to the midline ectodermal fusion during embryogenesis. They may be found on the penis, scrotum, or perineum.

Etiology: although MRC of the penis have been widely reported, their etiopathogenesis is obscure. They are thought to arise from embryologic developmental defects of the male urethra.

Epidemiology: MRC are a rare condition.

Clinical appearance: they occur as solitary, freely movable nodules on the ventral surface of the penis. In general, the lesion is asymptomatic and does not interfere with urinary or sexual function. Trauma and infection are possible complications.

Clinical course: most lesions are present at birth but remain undetectable until adolescence or adulthood.

Diagnosis: it is clinical. Videodermatoscopy may be helpful in the differentiation between cysts and canals of the median raphe of the penis, showing in the latter case the presence of a tract connecting cystic lesions.

Therapy: unless the cysts are small and asymptomatic, excision is usually recommended.

Suggested Reading

Cardoso R, Freitas JD, Reis JP, Tellechea O (2005) Median raphe cyst of the penis. Dermatol Online J 11:37

Lacarrubba F, Tedeschi A, Francesconi L, Micali G (2010) Canal versus cysts of the penile median raphe: advancing diagnostic methods using videodermatoscopy. Pediatr Dermatol 27:667-9

Micali G, Lacarrubba F (2011) Augmented diagnostic capability using videodermatoscopy on selected infectious and non-infectious penile growths. Int J Dermatol 50:1501-5

Navarro HP, Lopez PC, Ruiz J et al (2009) Median raphe cyst. Report of two cases and literature review. Arch Esp Urol 62:585-9

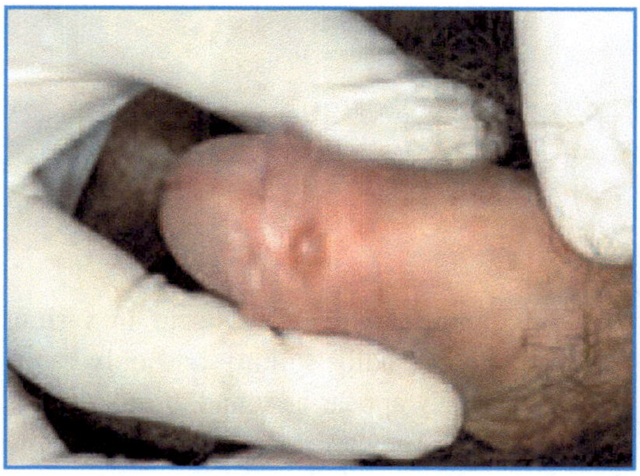

Fig. 9.4 Translucent and round nodule located in the midline of the ventral surface of penis

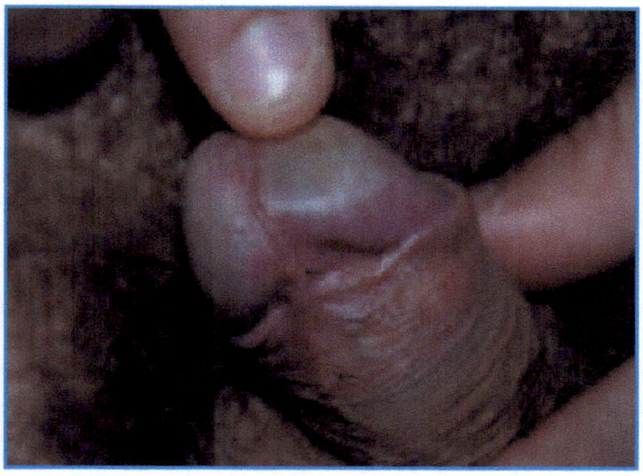

Fig. 9.5 Translucent and raised papules along the ventral surface of penis

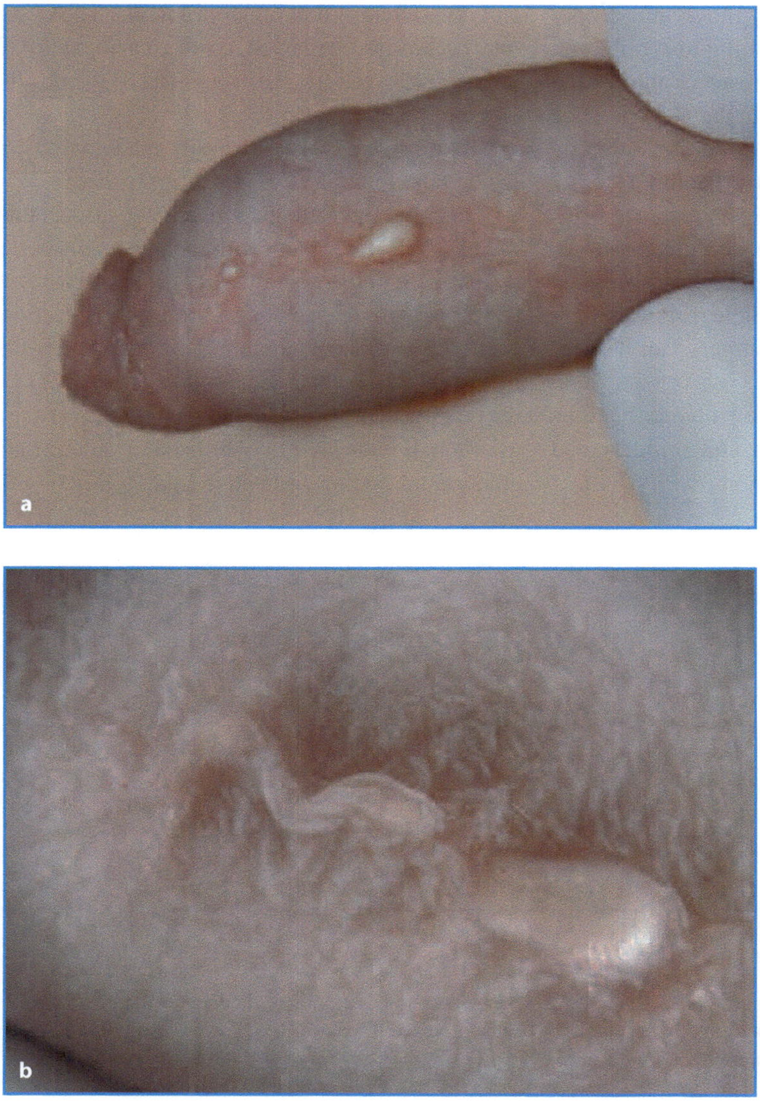

Fig. 9.6 Median raphe canal. a Smooth, soft, and yellowish papules located in the midline of the ventral surface of penis in a child. b Videodermatoscopy (X30) reveals the presence of a translucent tract connecting and encompassing the three lesions, allowing a definitive diagnosis of median raphe canal

Epidermoid Cysts

Definition: Epidermoid Cysts (EC) are small bumps that can develop beneath the skin of face, neck, trunk, and sometimes genital area. Epidermoid glands arise from the cells that make up the outer layers of skin (epidermal). True sebaceous cysts arising from the sebaceous glands are less common.

Etiology: some epidermal or follicular cells close to the skin surface may move into deeper parts of the skin while continuing to proliferate. These cells may arrange themselves into round structures, gathering the keratin that they produce and that would normally be released on the top layer of the skin. The keratin becomes soggy and turns into a toothpaste-like substance. Epidermoid/sebaceous cysts may be congenital or acquired. In the etiology of acquired cysts, trauma (damage to a hair follicle, rupture of sebaceous gland) or previous surgery can be considered as causes.

Epidemiology: EC can affect anyone, but they are most common in young and middle-aged adults. Penile EC are uncommon.

Clinical appearance: EC occur in various sizes, they are usually solitary and only rarely multifocal. They appear as round, usually small, mobile bumps. They are usually white or yellow, though people with darker skin may have pigmented cysts. Lesions may be asymptomatic, but rupture may result in significant discomfort.

Clinical course: epidermoid cysts are benign and do not cause functional problems. The cysts may became red, inflamed, ruptured and painful if infected. Very rarely, they may lead to the development of skin cancer .

Diagnosis: it is usually easily made based on the clinical findings.

Therapy: indications for treatment are secondary cyst infection, pain on intercourse, cosmetic concerns, or obstruction of the urinary tract. A course of antibiotics will usually clear an infection if it occurs. Simple complete excision followed by primary closure has generally been regarded as the best treatment procedure. To minimize scarring, a carbon dioxide laser may be used to vaporize an epidermoid cyst on a sensitive area.

Suggested Reading

Saini P, Mansoor MN, Jalali S, Sharma A (2010) Penile epidermal inclusion cyst. Indian J Pediatr 77:815-6

Singh S, Kaur T (2011) Epidermoid cyst of penis. Indian J Dermatol Venereol Leprol 77:627

Suwa M, Takeda M, Bilim V, Takahashi K (2000) Epidermoid cyst of the penis: a case report and review of the literature. Int J Urol 7:431-3

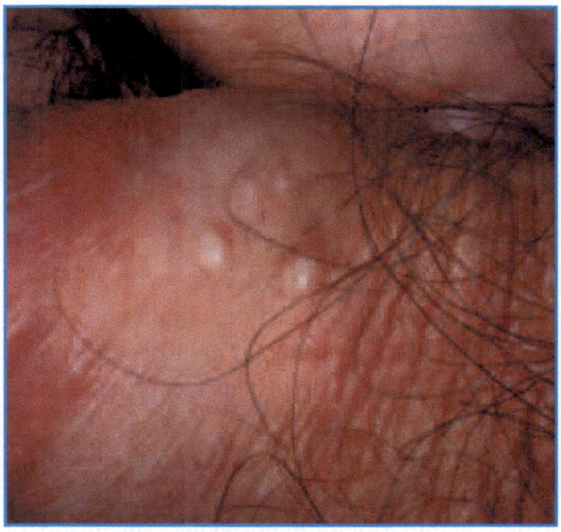

Fig. 9.7 Yellowish and round papules on the shaft

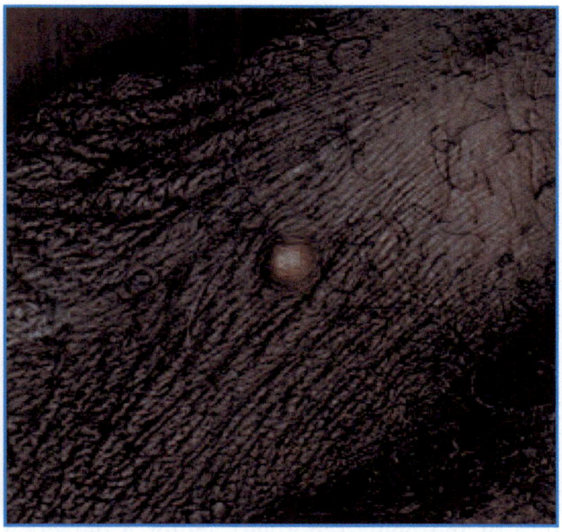

Fig. 9.8 Brownish and round nodule of the shaft in an Afro-American patient

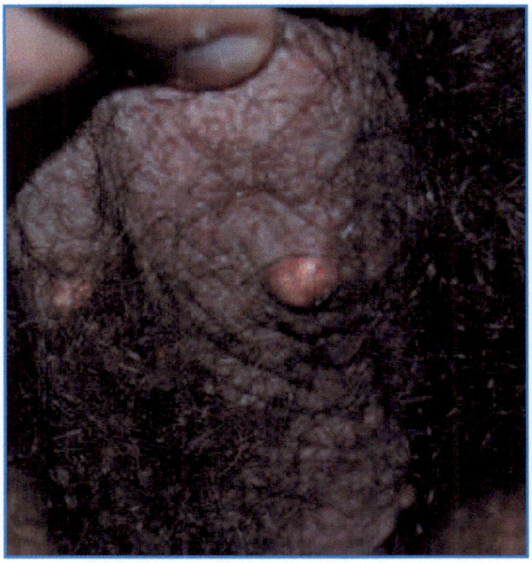

Fig. 9.9 Yellowish nodules on the scrotum

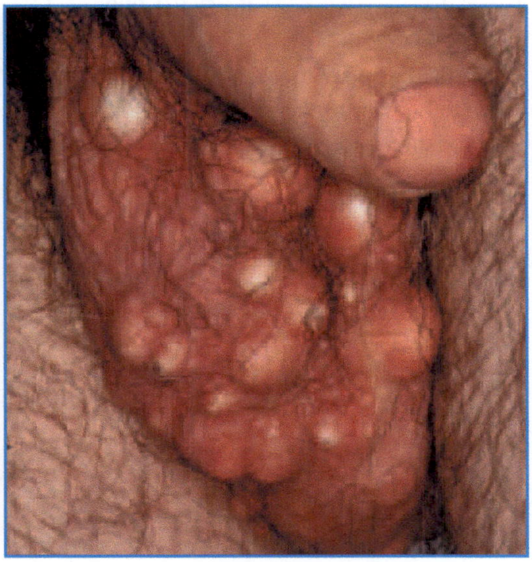

Fig. 9.10 Multiple, confluent, and yellowish nodules on the scrotum

Hypospadia

Definition: Hypospadia (H) is an abnormality of anterior urethral and penile development in which an abnormal urethral opening is ectopically located on the ventral penis. The urethral opening may be located as far down as the scrotum or perineum, extending up to the navicular fossa. H is often associated with a ventral curvature of the penis (chordee) and/or a defective ventral foreskin.

Etiology: several etiologies for H have been suggested, including genetic, endocrine, and environmental factors.

Epidemiology: it is a relatively frequent disorder of the external genitalia (1-8/1,000 newborn boys).

Clinical appearance: three anatomic variants of H are known: of the glans (the urinary meatus is on the underside of the glans), of the shaft (the urinary meatus is in the middle of the penis), and of the scrotum (the embryologic fusion of the genital swellings is lost and a urethral opening at the level of the scrotum remains).

Clinical course: hypospadias are usually asymptomatic. Distal hypospadias without curvature do not cause any functional limitations. Proximal hypospadias can impair control of the urine stream. An accompanying curvature can hinder sexual intercourse.

Diagnosis: it is made from a thorough knowledge of past medical history and physical examination. Familiarity for hypospadias, any history or comorbidity, and a physical assessment focusing on the position of the meatus, glans configuration, skin coverage, and chordee are important steps in patient evaluation.

Therapy: distal hypospadias may not require surgical repair and may simply be managed with observation. In proximal hypospadias, early corrective surgery is the appropriate treatment. However, hypospadias are surgically treated for functional reasons (prevention of urination from a standing position, substenotic meatus), sexual reasons (correction of infertility due to impotence from penile curvature), and aesthetic reasons (the altered penile appearance may cause severe psychological problems).

Suggested Reading

Brouwers MM, van der Zanden LF, de Gier RP et al (2010) Hypospadias: risk factor patterns and different phenotypes. BJU Int 105:254-62

Kalfa N, Philibert P, Baskin LS, Sultan C (2011) Hypospadias: interactions between environment and genetics. Mol Cell Endocrinol 335:89-95

Kraft KH, Shukla AR, Canning DA (2010) Hypospadias. Urol Clin North Am 37:167-81

Van Der Zanden LF, Van Rooij IA, Feitz WF et al (2012) Aetiology of hypospadias: a systematic review of genes and environment. Hum Reprod Update 18:260-83

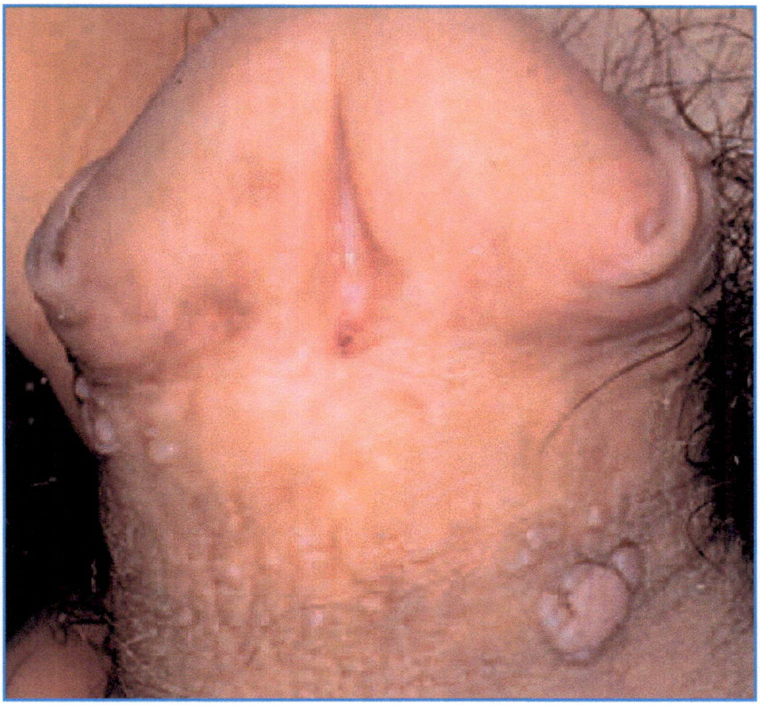

Fig. 9.11 The urethral meatus is on the underside of the glans; this patient also presented with multiple warts

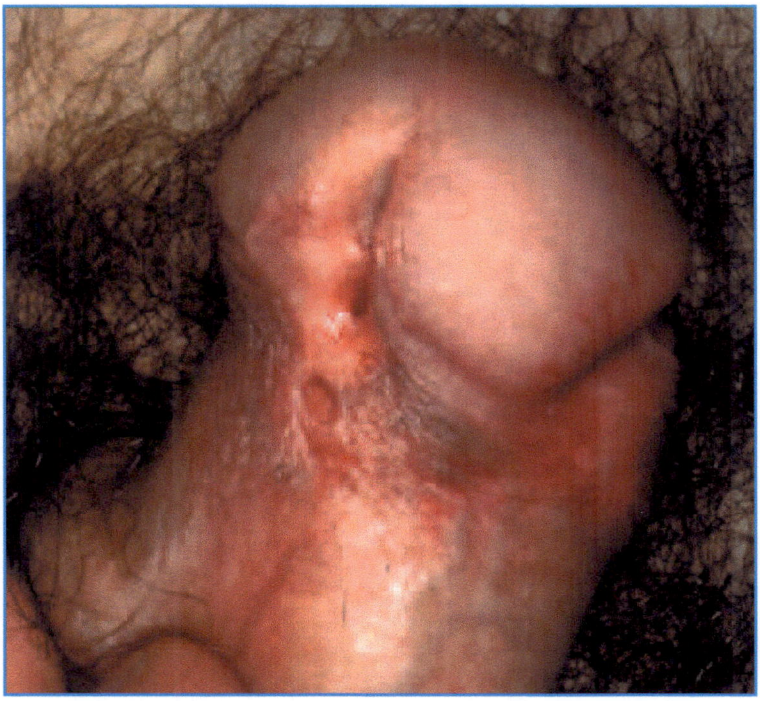

Fig. 9.12 Associated diffuse erythema due to impaired control of the urine stream

10 Miscellaneous Disorders

Marco Cusini, Stefano Ramoni, Anna Elisa Verzì,
and Franco Dinotta

M. Cusini (✉)
Center for Sexually Transmitted Diseases
Dermatology Unit
Dipartimento di Anestesiologia, Terapia Intensiva e Scienze Dermatologiche
Fondazione IRCCS Ca' Granda
Ospedale Maggiore Policlinico, Milan, Italy
e-mail: m.cusini@policlinico.mi.it

G. Micali et al., *Atlas of Male Genital Disorders*,
DOI: 10.1007/978-88-470-2787-9_10, © Springer-Verlag Italia 2013

Phimosis (Acquired)

Definition: phimosis is the inability to retract the narrowed prepuce (distal foreskin) behind the glans penis in uncircumcised men.

Etiology: the narrowing or constriction of the foreskin is normal during early infancy. Pathologic phimosis is commonly acquired as a result of poor hygiene, recurrent episodes of bacterial infection (balanitis or balanoposthitis), chronic inflammation with loss of skin elasticity (elderly individuals), lichen sclerosus of the foreskin, and diabetes.

Epidemiology: the prevalence of adhesions between prepuce and glans are age dependent: 58% after 1 year, and 10-35% after 3 years of age. In uncircumcised males, a prevalence of 8% has been reported at 6 years, and of 1% at 16 years of age for true phimosis (with scarring).

Clinical appearance: it is characterized by scarring and obstruction of the opening of the foreskin (preputial stenosis). The skin appears thickened, whitish, and stiff.

Clinical course: complications of phimosis include balanitis, posthitis, paraphimosis, and penile carcinoma. Proper foreskin hygiene, including gentle retraction and cleansing during bathing, helps to prevent pathologic foreskin conditions.

Diagnosis: it is diagnosed during physical examination.

Therapy: a nonretractable foreskin in a prepubescent child is not a disease and requires no treatment. Once phimosis is diagnosed, the available treatments include topical corticosteroids, manual retraction, preputioplasty and circumcision. Conservative treatments should be tried in the first instance and surgery used as the treatment in more advanced phimosis. The success rate of conservative therapy is around 75–90%. Preputioplasty consists of a dorsal, longitudinal incision through the constrictive band of the foreskin. This procedure has less morbidity than circumcision, and allows the prepuce to be retained. Complete (radical) or incomplete (prepuce sparing) circumcision is the cornerstone of advanced phimosis treatment.

Suggested Reading

Bromage SJ, Crump A, Pearce I (2008) Phimosis as a presenting feature of diabetes. BJU Int 101:338-40

Hayashi Y, Kojima Y, Mizuno K, Kohri K (2011) Prepuce: phimosis, paraphimosis, and circumcision. ScientificWorldJournal 11:289-301

Reddy S, Jain V, Dubey M et al (2012) Local steroid therapy as the first-line treatment for boys with symptomatic phimosis - a long-term prospective study. Acta Paediatr 101:e130-3

Shankar KR, Rickwood AM (1999) The incidence of phimosis in boys. BJU Int 84:101-2

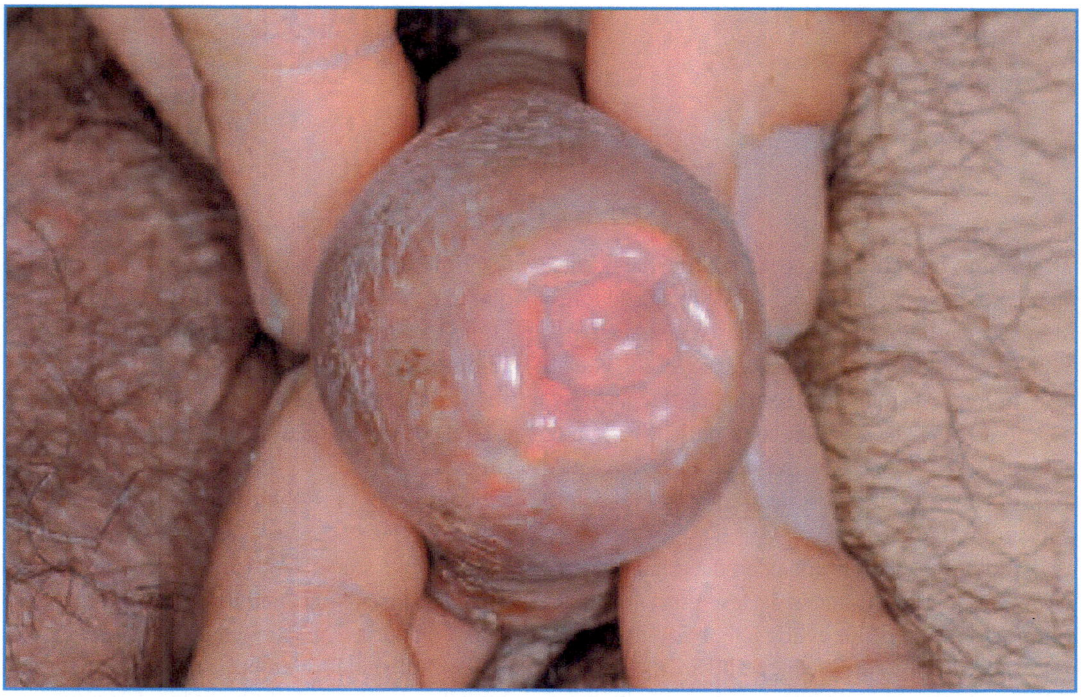

Fig. 10.1 Constriction of the foreskin opening in a patient with lichen sclerosus; the penile skin appears thickened and sclerotic

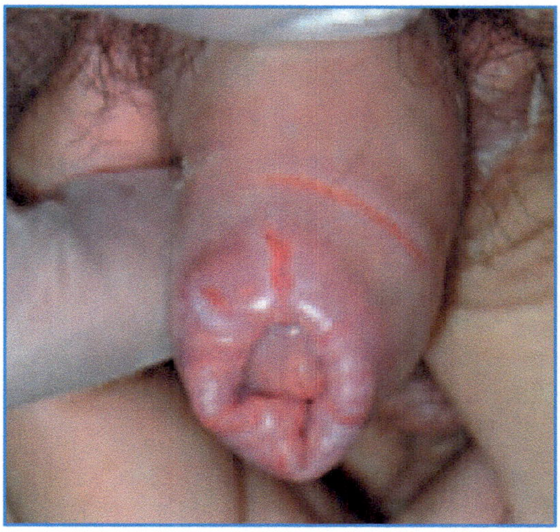

Fig. 10.2 Phimosis and fissuring in candidiasis

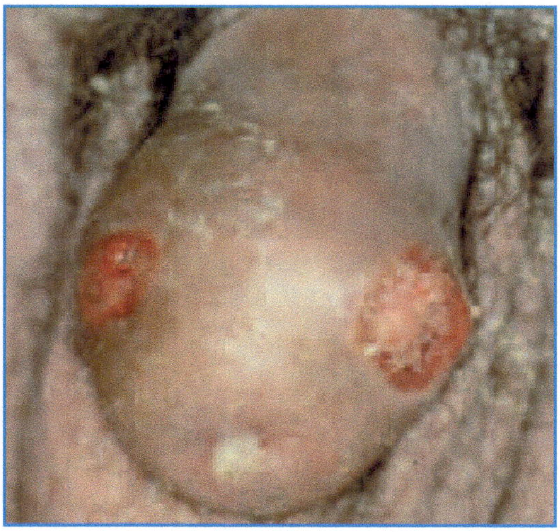

Fig. 10.3 Phimosis resulting from massive neoplastic infiltration of the foreskin from squamous cell carcinoma of the glans ("window sign")

Paraphimosis

Definition: paraphimosis is a condition that occurs in uncircumcised patients when the retracted foreskin narrows below the glans, constricting the lymphatic drainage and causing swelling of the glans.

Etiology: it frequently results from a partially phimotic foreskin that has been pulled back and not released. It can also frequently occur in patients with a urethral catheter in place and the foreskin retracted.

Epidemiology: it is considered a relatively uncommon condition, and it is less common than phimosis. It can occur at any age, but it is mostly observed during adolescence and in the elderly who need frequent catheterizations and who have a history of poor hygiene or recurrent bacterial infections.

Clinical appearance: the glans is erythematous and swollen, and the retracted foreskin is trapped behind it. The condition may be very painful.

Clinical course: when untreated, it can progress to ischemia of the glans and to eventual gangrene.

Diagnosis: it is diagnosed during physical examination.

Therapy: since hypoxia from reduced blood flow can cause tissue death (necrosis), paraphimosis is considered a medical emergency and requires immediate treatment. An initial attempt at manual reduction should be made. Circumcision is recommended after treatment to prevent recurrences.

Suggested Reading

Dubin J, Davis JE (2011) Penile emergencies. Emerg Med Clin North Am 29:485-99

Hayashi Y, Kojima Y, Mizuno K, Kohri K (2011) Prepuce: phimosis, paraphimosis, and circumcision. ScientificWorldJournal 11:289-301

Kessler CS, Bauml J (2009) Non-traumatic urologic emergencies in men: a clinical review. West J Emerg Med 10:281-7

Little B, White M (2005) Treatment options for paraphimosis. Int J Clin Pract 59:591-3

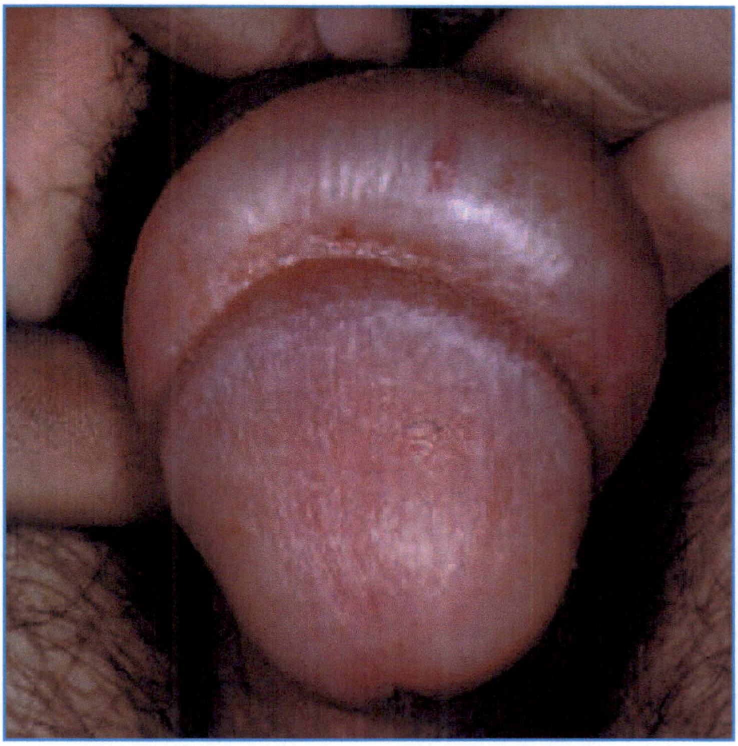

Fig. 10.4 The foreskin, trapped behind the glans, is erythematous and swollen

Synechiae

Definition: synechiae are remnants of the fused layers between the glans and prepuce. They are also known as balanopreputial membranes or balanopreputial laminae. Confusingly, the term "synechiae" is also used to refer to skin-bridges.

Etiology: they are linked to developmental abnormalities. Acquired forms may be due to chronic inflammation resulting in scarring.

Epidemiology: they are unusual.

Clinical appearance: synechiae appear as triangular skin folds located in the lower portion of the glans penis and attached between the inner foreskin and the glans.

Clinical course: balanopreputial adhesions are common among children. Eventually, they dissolve naturally, and break down following foreskin retraction and intermittent erections. In case of persistence, development of lichen sclerosus, or even in situ or invasive squamous cell carcinoma, is possible.

Diagnosis: they are visible during physical examination.

Therapy: by the teenage years they should have completely disappeared. Rarely, they have to be removed by a stretching technique or surgery, called preputioplasty.

Suggested Reading

Kumar P, Deb M, Das K (2009) Preputial adhesions – a misunderstood entity. Indian J Pediatr 76:829-32
Kolehmainen M, Taskinen S, Ossi L (2010) Foreskin surgery. Duodecim 126:75-83
Gracely-Kilgore KA (1984) Penile adhesion: the hidden complication of circumcision. Nurse Pract 9:22-4

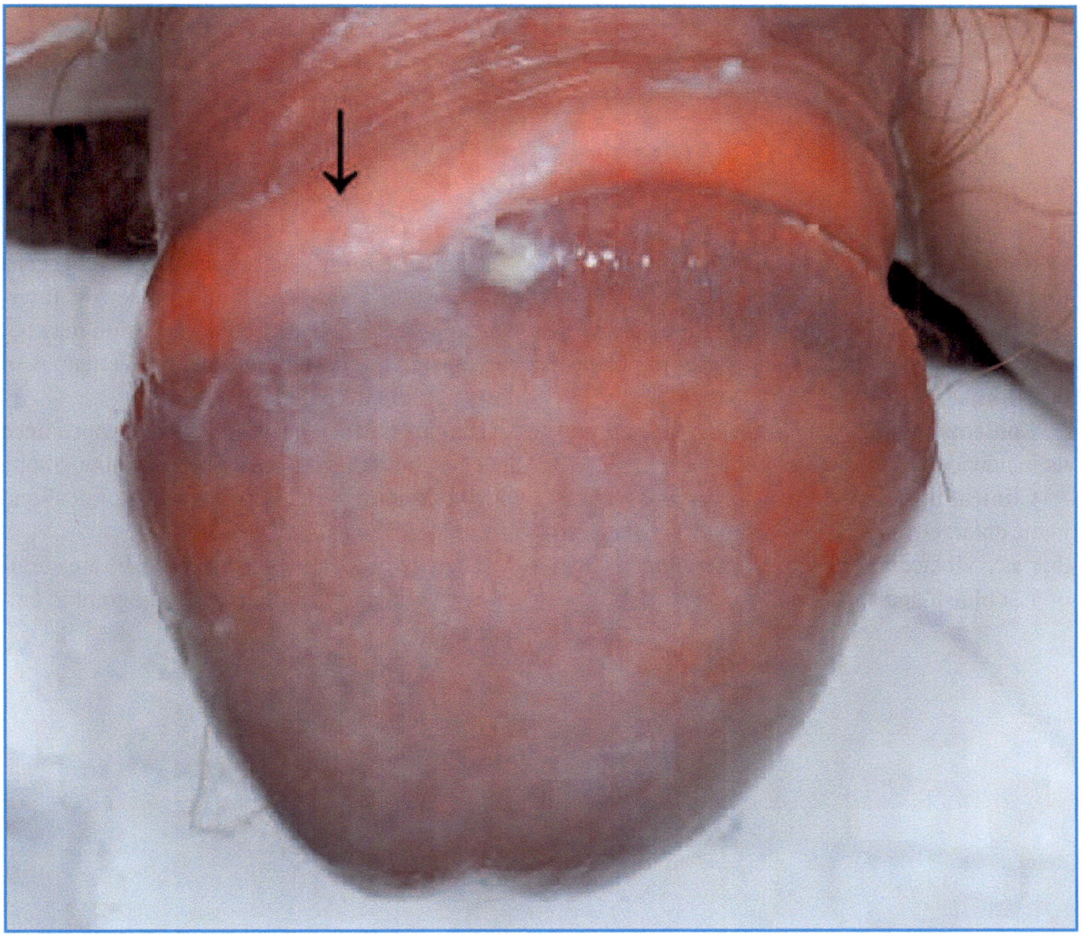

Fig. 10.5 Adhesions between the inner foreskin and the glans (*arrow*); the onset of squamous cell carcinoma at this level is likely

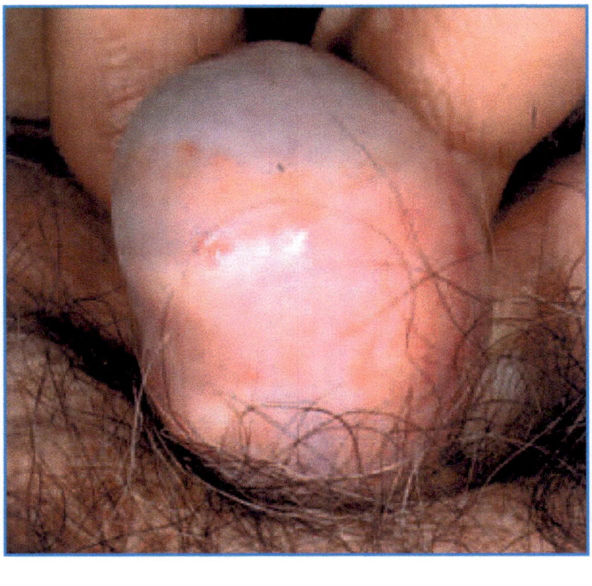

Fig. 10.6 Disappearance of the coronal sulcus in a patient with genital lichen sclerosus

Phlebectasia

Definition: phlebectasia is an abnormal dilatation of the veins of the penis.

Etiology: local anatomic alterations are typically implicated as the primary causes of phlebectasia formation.

Epidemiology: the condition is rather unusual; its incidence increases after puberty.

Clinical appearance: it appears as asymptomatic enlarged vessels on foreskin or on glans, either as a violaceous, raised, and serpiginous tract or as a bluish and soft nodule.

Clinical course: the presence of phlebectasia has no significant functional impact on intercourse. Occasionally, vascular occlusion may occur causing the development of erythematous or dark painful swellings.

Diagnosis: anamnesis and clinical appearance are enough for diagnosis. Doppler ultrasonography may be used to better define the anatomical and physiological features.

Therapy: recommended techniques are surgical resection and percutaneous radiographic embolization.

Suggested Reading

Balato N, Montesano M, Lembo G (1985) Acquired phlebectasia of the glans penis. J Am Acad Dermatol 13(5 Pt 1):824-6

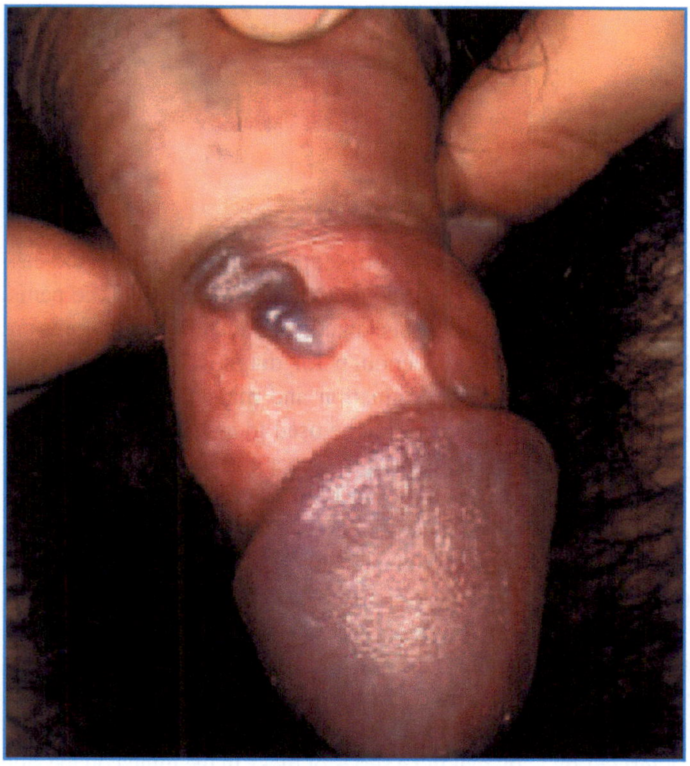

Fig. 10.7 Violaceous, raised, and serpiginous tract within the inner foreskin

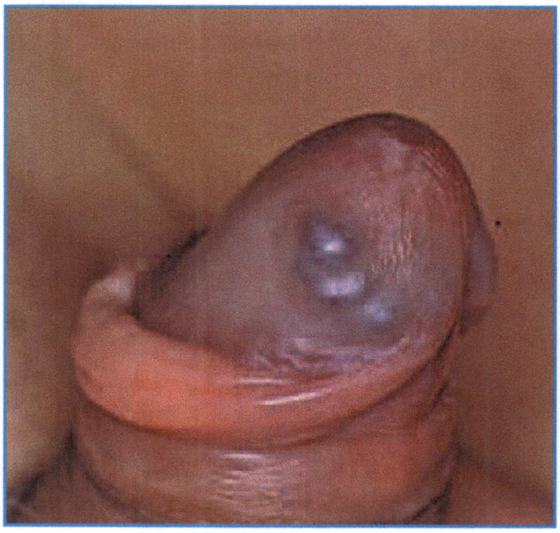

Fig. 10.8 Bluish and soft nodules on the glans

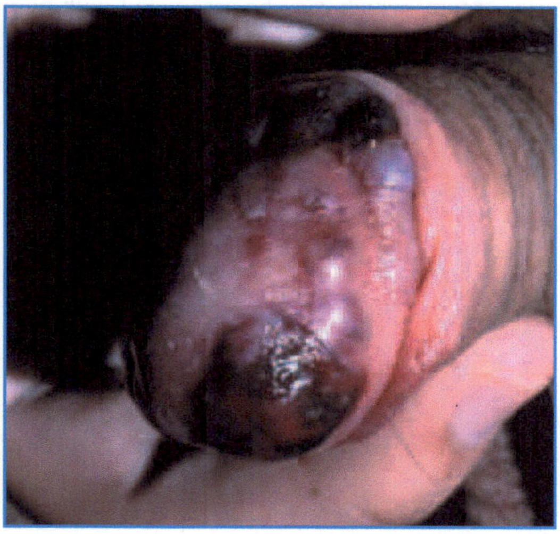

Fig. 10.9 Reddish to black nodules on the glans, with evidence of vascular occlusion

Induratio Penis Plastica

Definition: Induratio Penis Plastica (IPP), also known as Peyronie's disease, is a chronic fibrotic process involving the penis.

Etiology: its cause is still not fully explained, although some evidence suggests that repeated microtrauma, hormonal dysfunction, metabolic disorders (diabetes, gout), and a general fibroplastic disposition may play a role. It may occur in association with similar lumps of fibrous tissue in the palms of the hands (Dupuytren's contracture), nodules in the ears, and retroperitoneal fibrosis.

Epidemiology: IPP accounts for 0.3-0.7% of all urologic disorders. It occurs most often in the fourth to sixth decades of life, and occasionally in men less than 20 years old.

Clinical appearance: IPP is characterized by palpable nodules in the region of the tunica albuginea enclosing the corpora cavernosa and the penile septum, which may be associated with pain and deformity on erection and a variable degree of erectile dysfunction.

Clinical course: patients usually have increasingly painful erection and deviation of the penis.

Diagnosis: anamnesis and clinical features are generally enough for diagnosis. A penile ultrasound examination and magnetic resonance angiography may be used to assess the localization of plaques and to detect possible calcifications.

Therapy: various treatments have been suggested, such as estrogens, vitamin E, potassium para-aminobenzoate, local infiltration of steroids, and radiation therapy. Whatever treatment is given, in many cases the discomfort ceases and the deformity reduces spontaneously. When the condition is particularly painful, or the angulation of the penis prevents intercourse, the penis can be straightened by making a series of tucks in the tunica on the side opposite to the plaque. The patient should be made aware that some loss of penile shaft length may occur. Surgical treatment (excision of the plaques and tissue replacement) has been considered in advanced stages of the disease.

Suggested Reading

Abdel-Hamid IA, Anis T (2011) Peyronie's disease: perspectives on therapeutic targets. Expert Opin Ther Targets 15:913-29

Larsen SM, Levine LA (2012) Review of non-surgical treatment options for Peyronie's disease. Int J Impot Res 24:1-10

Ralph D, Gonzalez-Cadavid N, Mirone V et al (2010) The management of Peyronie's disease: evidence-based 2010 guidelines. J Sex Med 7:2359-74

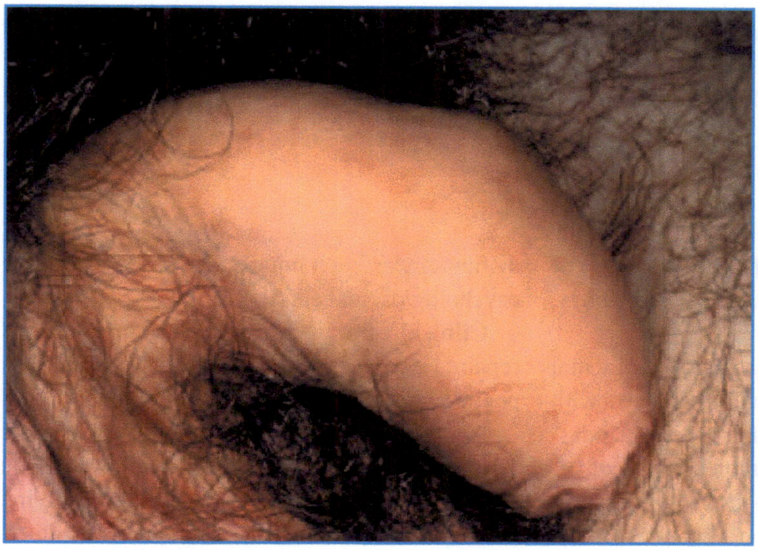

Fig. 10.10 Palpable nodules of the shaft which may be associated with pain and deformity on erection

Traumatic and Self-Induced Lesions

Definition: traumatic and self-induced lesions of the external genitalia are disorders caused by physical or chemical injuries.

Etiology: they are mainly due to accidental penetrating or blunt mechanical traumas, with about 10% of cases consequent to burns and industrial accidents. The most common etiology of penile fracture is a direct blow to the erect penis during intercourse or masturbation. Fracture is a tear in the tunica albuginea of the penis. Erection thins out the tunica and makes it more susceptible to injury. Neurotic and psychotic excoriations are associated with depression and psychoses.

Epidemiology: traumatic injuries are common. Self-induced lesions are rarely seen.

Clinical appearance: the common presentation of penile fracture is in a patient who reports a "cracking" or "popping" sound, immediate pain, rapid detumescence, penile swelling and penile deviation away from the injury. Associated urethral injury occurs in 15-22% of fractures. Unless there is blood at the meatus, hematuria is present, or voiding is difficult. Frequently, self-induced excoriations or ulcers have a linear border or a geometric pattern. In addition to cosmetic and functional disfigurement, such injuries can have devastating psychological and emotional effects.

Clinical course: corporal injuries that are not repaired early can result in erectile dysfunction, penile scarring, curvature, pain and infection.

Diagnosis: location of the fracture can often be identified on physical examination by a palpable defect in the tunica, focal tenderness, or overlying hematoma with contralateral penile deflection. Cavernosography can accurately diagnose and localize the rupture site. However, this procedure is rarely indicated because it is invasive, time-consuming and difficult to interpret. Recurrent or necrotic lesions without evident cause should always raise suspicion of self-inflicted traumas.

Therapy: the main goal is to prevent penile deformity or erectile dysfunction. Management involves prompt exploration, hematoma evacuation and primary repair of the tunica albuginea with absorbable suture. Treatment of neurotic or psychotic excoriations is based on the administration of antidepressants, and should include psychiatric consultation. Local supportive measures with topical antibiotics and protective dressing may be helpful.

Suggested Reading

Al-Shaiji TF, Amann J, Brock GB (2009) Fractured penis: diagnosis and management. J Sex Med 6:3231-40

Koifman L, Barros R, Júnior RA et al (2010) Penile fracture: diagnosis, treatment and outcomes of 150 patients. Urology 76:1488-92

Shenfeld OZ, Gnessin E (2011) Management of urogenital trauma: state of the art. Curr Opin Urol 21:449-54

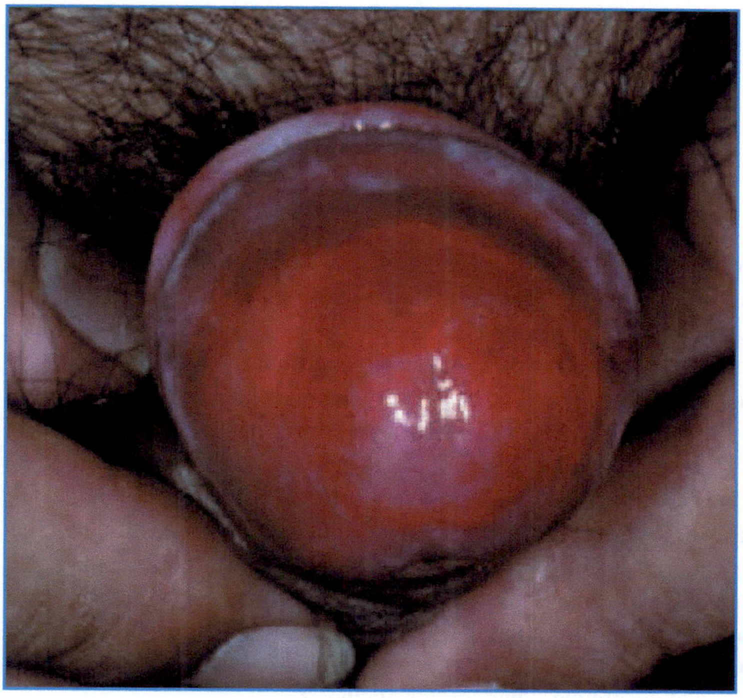

Fig. 10.11 Diffuse erosion of the glans caused by a burn

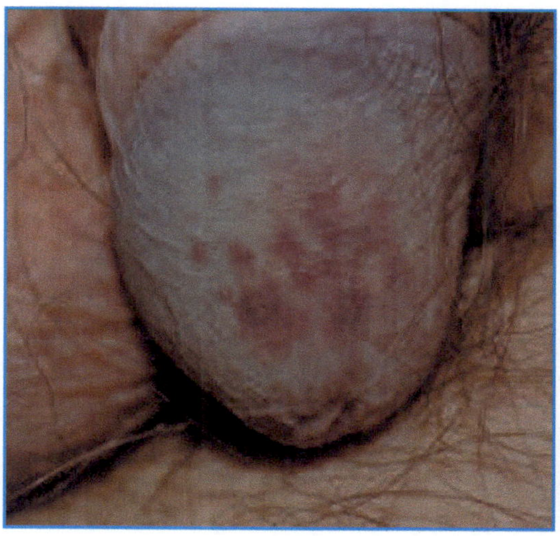

Fig. 10.12 Multiple hemorrhagic lesions on the glans

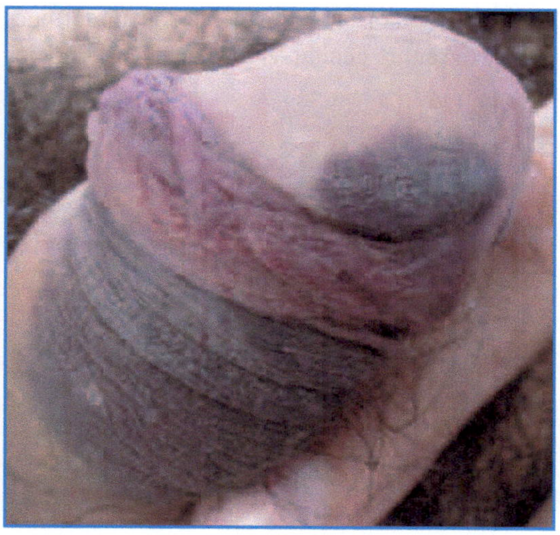

Fig. 10.13 Extensive hematoma involving the glans, foreskin, and shaft

Tattoos

Definition: tattoos are cutaneous pigmentations from exogenous coloured material knowingly (decorative tattoos) or accidentally (accidental tattoos) introduced permanently into the skin. Medical tattoos are commonly used to delineate permanent landmarks for radiation therapy and are performed by a physician.

Etiology: decorative tattoos are made for aesthetic, religious or cultural reasons. Accidental tattoos are the consequence of contamination through injury, for example during road accidents.

Epidemiology: decorative tattoos are globally widespread, notably in young people.

Clinical appearance: in the case of decorative tattoos, the clinical appearance varies according to the colours and designs used. Accidental tattoos are greyish or black and the design is undefined. Nearly the entire genital region can be tattooed, including the shaft and the head of the penis, the skin of the scrotum and the pubic region. Some men have incorporated genital tattooing into the creation of a tattoo design in such a way that the penis becomes a part of the overall design motif.

Clinical course: complications in the case of decorative tattoos are rare and they are characterized by allergic reaction to different pigments, foreign body reactions, and transmission of infectious diseases, such as HIV, syphilis, and hepatitis. Rarely, Koebner phenomenon may occur in patients with lichen planus, psoriasis, or vitiligo.

Diagnosis: anamnesis and clinical features are enough for diagnosis.

Therapy: they can be removed by lasertherapy. Surgical treatment should be avoided and reserved to very small lesions because of the risk of scarring.

Suggested Reading

Adatto MA, Halachmi S, Lapidoth M (2011) Tattoo removal. Curr Probl Dermatol 42:97-110

Angulo JC, García-Díez M, Martínez M (2011) Phallic decoration in paleolithic art: genital scarification, piercing and tattoos. J Urol 186:2498-503

Raulin C, Schönermark MP, Greve B, Werner S (1998) Q-switched ruby laser treatment of tattoos and benign pigmented skin lesions: a critical review. Ann Plast Surg 41:555-65

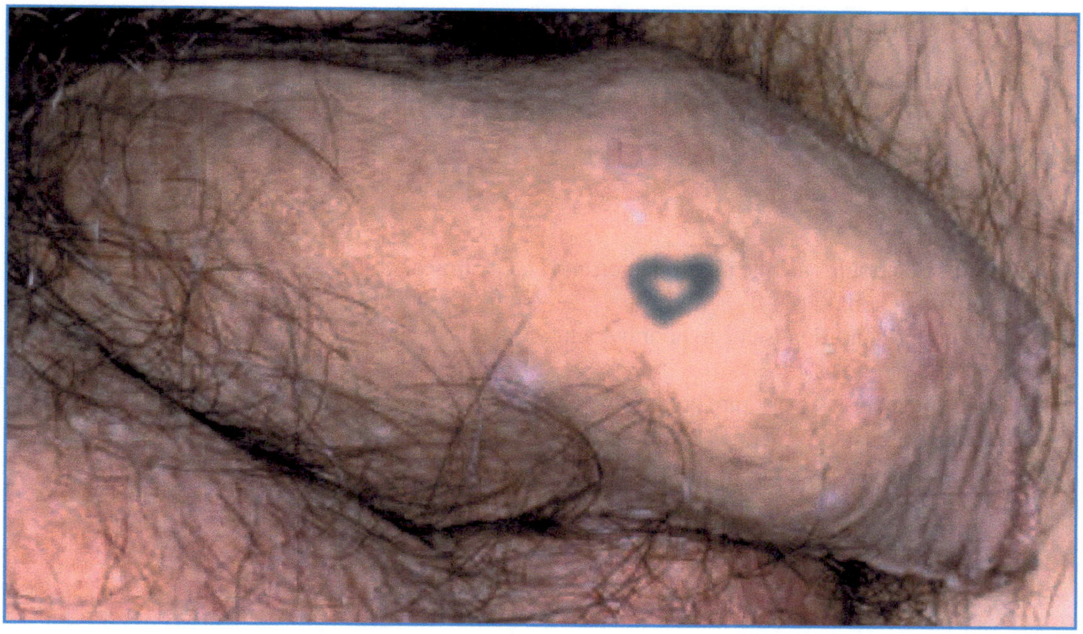

Fig. 10.14 Decorative tattoo: bluish “heart” in a patient with lichen planus

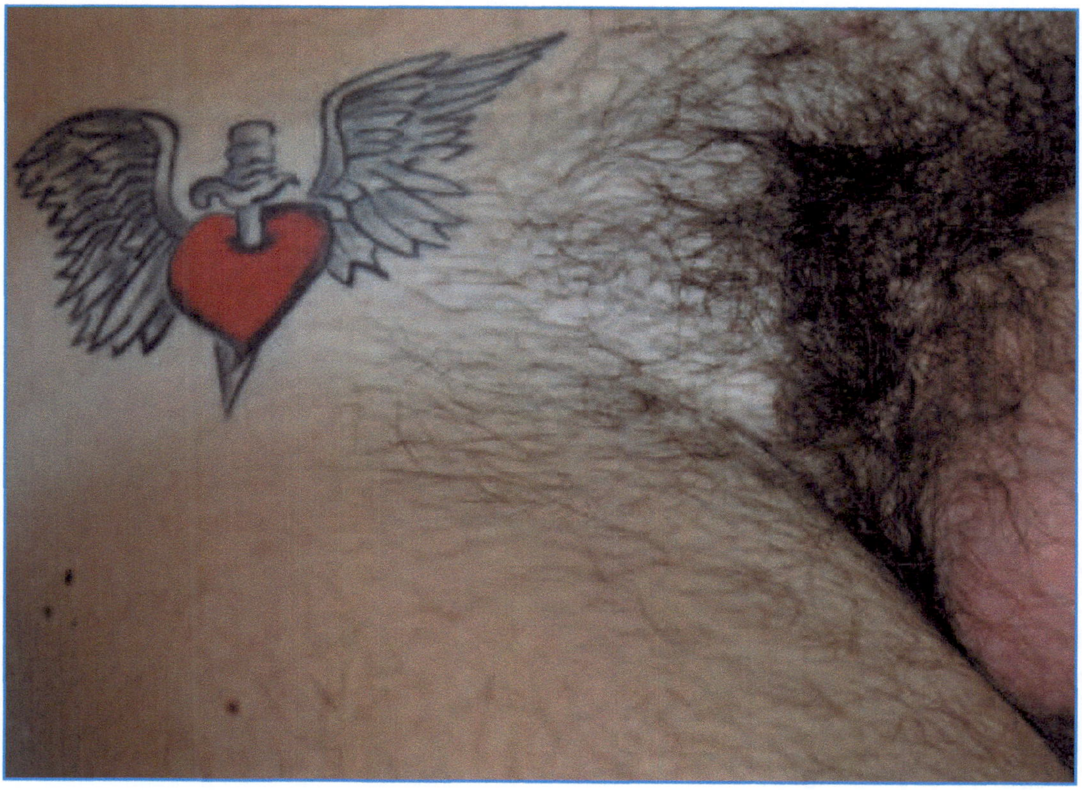

Fig. 10.15 Decorative tattoo of the pubis

Smegmoliths

Definition: smegmoliths are the accumulation and concretion of smegma.

Etiology: this condition is due to poor hygiene and/or chronic phimosis.

Epidemiology: it is a very rare condition.

Clinical appearance: smegma assumes a consistency similar to clay and it is difficult to remove.

Clinical course: since they are associated with chronic balanitis, smegmoliths represent a risk factor for the onset of squamous cell carcinoma.

Diagnosis: easily based on clinical observation.

Therapy: it consists of mechanical removal after application of topical emollients.

Suggested Reading

Braun O (1951) A case of smegmoliths. Dermatol Wochenschr 123:539-40

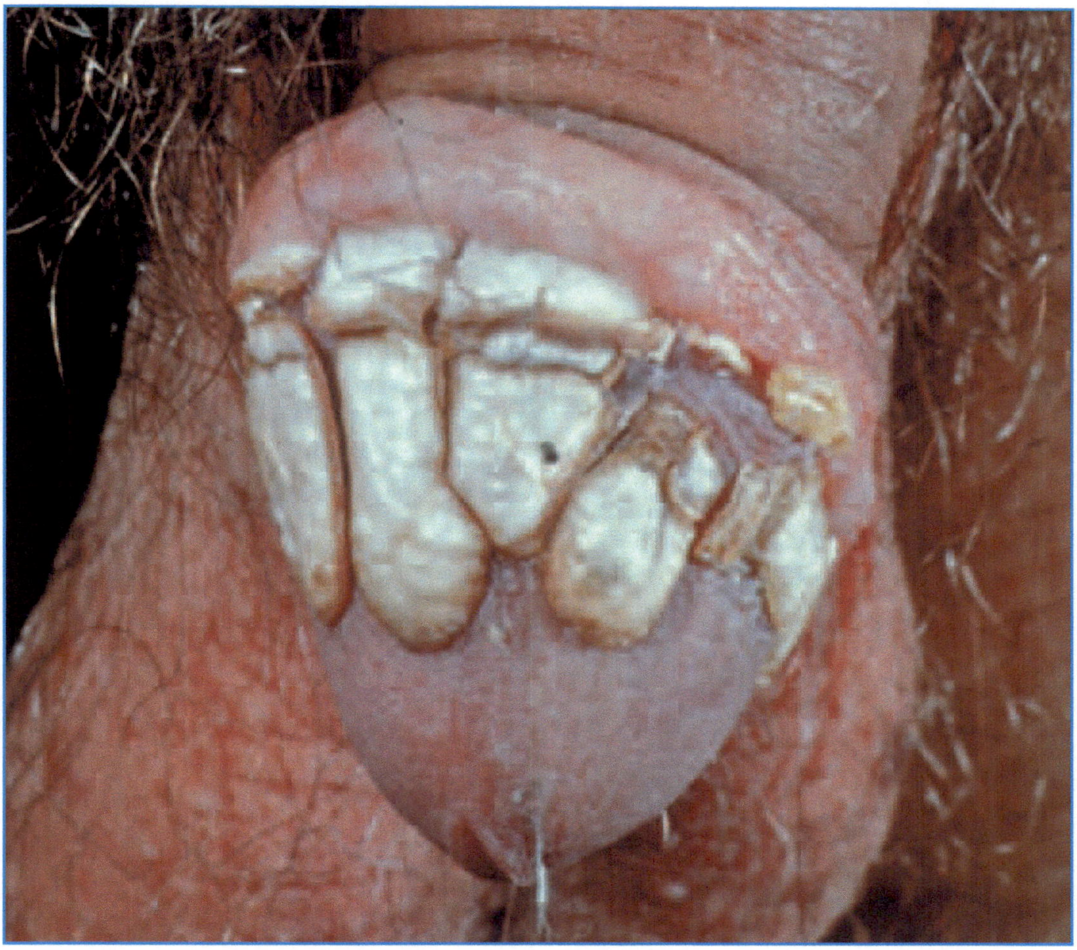

Fig. 10.16 Concretions of smegma with hardness similar to clay

MIX
Papier aus verantwortungsvollen Quellen
Paper from responsible sources
FSC® C105338

If you have any concerns about our products,
you can contact us on
ProductSafety@springernature.com

In case Publisher is established outside the EU,
the EU authorized representative is:
Springer Nature Customer Service Center GmbH
Europaplatz 3, 69115 Heidelberg, Germany

Printed by Libri Plureos GmbH
in Hamburg, Germany